3—

D0872344

A Change
of Heart

A Change of Heart

A MEMOIR

Claire Sylvia *with*
William Novak

FOREWORD BY

BERNIE SIEGEL, M.D.

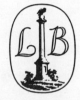

LITTLE, BROWN AND COMPANY

A *Little, Brown* Book

First published in Great Britain in 1997
by Little, Brown and Company

Copyright © 1997 by Claire Sylvia and William Novak
Foreword copyright © 1997 by Bernie Siegel, M.D.

The author is grateful for permission to include the
following previously copyrighted material:
Excerpt from "Mother's Evening Prayer" from *Poems* by Mary Baker Eddy.
Reprinted by permission of The First Church of Christ,
Scientist, Boston, Massachusetts.

A CIP catalogue record for this book
is available from the British Library.

ISBN 0 316 88348 4

Printed and bound in Great Britain by
Clays Ltd, St Ives plc

Little, Brown and Company (UK)
Brettenham House
Lancaster Place
London WC2E 7EN

For Amara,

the joy of my life;

And in loving memory

of Tim

Contents

Note

To protect their privacy, I have changed the names of some of the individuals mentioned in this book, including the members of my donor's family and the transplant recipients who are quoted or written about in these pages.

Acknowledgments

William Novak and I want to recognize some of the many people who helped us along the way: Mary Ansaldo, John Brinduse, Isabella Clemente, Maureen Dezell, Larry Dosscy, Gail Eddy, Brendan Farrington, Patricia Garfield, Jim Gleason, Myrna Goldstein, Rick Ingrasci, Bob and Barbara Katz, Marilyn Kurtz, Ruth Levy, Mike Mattil, Marilyn Mazza, Taren Metson, Nancy Mulvehill, Pam Newton, Peter Ogden, Paul Pearsall, Elaine Rogers, Linda Russek, Terry Schraeder, Gary Schwartz, Rupert Sheldrake, Bernie Siegel, Walillian Tyson, Claire and George Vasios, and particularly Sheila Weiser.

We especially want to thank agent Ike Williams, whose early support and wise advice made this book possible; Robert Bosnak, who contributed many valuable hours and insights; and our editor, William Phillips, whose clear, consistent vision kept us on track.

I also wish to thank my friends and family members who were there when I needed them; Dr. John Baldwin and the wonderful staff at Yale–New Haven Hospital, and (again!) Gail Eddy; my fellow transplant recipients who shared their experiences; Bill and Linda Novak, who opened their hearts and their home to me; and Jerry Mulcahy, who remained at my side throughout this long and exciting project.

Finally, I am indebted to the family of Tim Lasalle for welcoming me, answering my questions, and — no small matter — saving my life.

Foreword

by BERNIE SIEGEL, M.D.

I know the truth of Claire Sylvia's remarkable story. I met her in the hospital shortly after her transplant, and we have stayed in touch since then.

While I can't necessarily explain the amazing things that have happened to Claire, I have no trouble believing them. That's why I enjoy speaking with astronomers and quantum physicists, who are continually dealing with mysterious and unexplained events. I look forward to the day when physicians, too, will be comfortable acknowledging and accepting the mysteries all around us.

That day is coming, and the signs are everywhere. People like Candace Pert, Joan Borysenko, and hundreds of others are exploring the frontiers of the mind body connection. In new journals like *Advances* and *Alternative Therapies,* scholars and thinkers are sharing new ways to understand the miracles of healing.

In San Francisco, a cardiologist named Randolph Byrd did a study on the effects of prayers in 393 coronary-care-unit patients. The group was randomly divided into two, half to be prayed for and half not, although neither the patients nor the administrators were told who was in which group. When the study was over, the prayed-for patients did statistically better.

Before this study was published, it was rejected by two major medical journals. That's unfortunate, because we need to open ourselves to all possibilities. If Dr. Byrd's article had been about a new drug that caused these kinds of results, it would have been published immediately.

Although doctors tend to shy away from metaphysics, science and the spirit don't have to be at odds. "The most beautiful experience we can have," wrote Einstein, "is the mysterious. It is the fundamental emotion which stands at the cradle of true art and true science."

Long before I met Claire, I began working with people who had serious illnesses. I found that about 15 to 20 percent of these patients, either consciously or unconsciously, wanted to die. Another, much larger group seemed most interested in pleasing the doctor. They took their pills faithfully, showed up for appointments, and generally did whatever the doctors advised — unless that advice included a radical change in their lifestyles.

The third group, another 15 to 20 percent, consisted of patients whom I call "exceptional." These people refuse to be victims. They educate themselves and become specialists in their own care. They don't hesitate to question their doctors, whom they regard as partners rather than authority figures. The key thing about exceptional patients is that they keep their power.

As you'll discover, Claire Sylvia was an exceptional patient — although in her case *patient* may be the wrong word. Patient, after all, implies a submissive sufferer who is willing to undergo whatever is necessary without speaking up or raising a little hell.

Exceptional patients don't act that way. They learn from others but they make their own decisions. They reach out and take chances, and if a particular treatment isn't working, they let it go and try something else.

Claire knew intuitively what many doctors are only now beginning to understand — that physical healing can be significantly helped by opening up the lines of communication between the mind and the body. One way of doing that is through our emotions: working through negative feelings such as hate and jealousy, and embracing positive emotions, such as love, acceptance, and forgiveness. Another way is to visualize the healing process taking place in our bodies, and Claire did that, too.

While our minds and our bodies communicate constantly with each other, most of this exchange occurs on an unconscious level. That's why I often advise patients to start recording their dreams, because the body cannot speak except by using symbols. Although dreams can be difficult to understand, Claire shows how important they can be in learning vital information that may not be accessible in other ways.

Meditation is another way of communicating with the inner self. Someone once said that prayer is talking, while meditation is listening. Actually, meditation is a way to temporarily *stop* listening to the pressures and distractions of everyday life in order to be attentive to our deeper thoughts and feelings. The physical benefits of meditation have been well documented by many researchers, including Dr. Herbert Benson, who showed Claire and many others how to meditate.

More than most of us, Claire Sylvia has experienced the mysterious. During the course of her exceptional journey, she has been willing to explore her psyche and to confront feelings that many of us repress. I hope you will open both your mind and your heart to her extraordinary story.

A Change
of Heart

One

The Deepest Breath

SEVERAL YEARS AGO, as I lay dying from a rare and fatal disease, my chest was sawed open and my heart and lungs were cut out of me. Into that hollow, scooped-out space, in a last-ditch effort to save my life, the doctors transplanted the heart and lungs of a young man who had just died in a motorcycle accident. In a sublime act of generosity and grace, his family had agreed to offer up this precious and singular gift to a total stranger.

Within hours of their decision, that young man's lungs were breathing in my body, while his heart was pumping my blood with a pace and a vitality I had never known before. When I awoke from the operation and returned to life, I assumed that my long journey was finally over.

In fact, it was just beginning.

Before long, I began to feel that I had received more than just new body parts. I began to wonder if my transplanted heart and lungs had somehow arrived with some of their own inclinations and memories. I had dreams and experienced changes that seemed to suggest that some aspects of my donor's spirit and personality now existed within me.

All my life I have been told that despite the protests of poets and the murmuring of mystics, the human heart is just a pump. An incredibly important pump, but only a pump, a monotonous, mandatory machine. According to this view, which is the accepted one in contemporary Western medicine, the heart contains no feelings and carries no wisdom, no knowledge, and no memories. And if one person's heart has previously resided in another person's body, that fact has no particular meaning or implication.

I used to believe these things, but today I know differently. Perhaps there are other ways to think of the heart. Maybe some of the many qualities that have been attributed to the heart over the centuries are more than metaphorical. Even today, in our enlightened, scientific era, we still refer to the heart when we discuss our feelings and our values. When love dies, or death strikes, we speak of being brokenhearted. We take heart and lose heart all the time. When we want to be demonstrative, we wear our heart on our sleeve; when a person is insensitive, we say he is heartless. Pure heart, aching heart, soft heart, valiant heart, noble heart, tender heart, understanding heart — the list goes on.

Could there possibly be some literal truth to these expressions? Even the most conservative cardiologist will acknowledge that the health and functioning of the heart are affected by certain emotional realities, including loneliness, depression, and alienation. And while it is commonly accepted that the mind and the body are deeply connected, we don't have nearly as many images or phrases pertaining to, say, the liver, the pancreas, or even the brain.

When I acquired a new heart, I also acquired a new rhythm, new impulses, new knowledge, and new questions. I found my-

self on a fascinating and mysterious journey that I hadn't anticipated and wasn't prepared for, a journey that was occasionally
frightening and sometimes euphoric. This adventure of discovery, and also of *self*-discovery, has forced me to look at life's
mysteries in a completely new way.

My journey began with the transplant, or perhaps earlier. But
I didn't fully understand that I was already on it until five
months after the operation, when I had an unusually vivid
dream:

> *It's a warm summer day. I'm standing in an open, outside
> place, a grassy field. With me is a young man who is tall, thin,
> and wiry, with sandy-colored hair. His name is Tim, and I
> think his last name may be Leighton, but I'm not sure. I think
> of him as Tim L. We're in a playful relationship, and we're
> good friends.*
>
> *The time has come for me to leave him, to join a performing
> group of acrobats. I start walking down a path, away from
> Tim. Suddenly I turn around, feeling that something remains
> unfinished between us. I walk back toward him to say goodbye.
> Tim watches me as I come closer, and he seems to be pleased
> that I am making my way back to him.*
>
> *We kiss — and as we do I inhale him into me. It feels like
> the deepest breath I have ever taken. And I know at that
> moment the two of us, Tim and I, will be together forever.*

I awoke from the dream exhilarated, as though I *had* just
taken the deepest breath of my life. I also felt that I had integrated the new heart and lungs within me.

Vivid dreams are not new to me. I pay close attention to the
images that come to me, and I record them regularly in my journal. Some of my dreams are enigmatic, a vague and complicated

puzzle to be mulled over later. But not this one. Until now, I had thought of my heart and lungs as having come from an anonymous stranger, an unknown young man whom I hadn't thought much about. But when this dream was over, something had changed. I woke up knowing — really *knowing* — that Tim L. was my donor and that some parts of his spirit and personality were now in me.

I was eager to verify this information. But how? The transplant program at Yale–New Haven Hospital, where I received my new heart and lungs, observed a strict code of confidentiality. The hospital officials maintained an ironclad rule that the donor's identity could never be revealed to the recipient. The same was true in reverse: the donor's family could never be told exactly who had received the various organs they had made available. Strictly speaking, I wasn't even supposed to know what little I did: that my donor was an eighteen-year-old boy, that he lived in Maine, and that he died on a motorcycle. I had heard these things from a nurse shortly after the operation.

The day after the dream, I called Gail Eddy, the transplant co-ordinator at Yale–New Haven, who had been enormously helpful to me before, during, and after the operation. I knew that Gail couldn't tell me who my donor was, but perhaps she would be willing to confirm the name of Tim L. from my dream. Assuming, of course, that my information was correct.

And at first I thought it was. When I told Gail about the dream and asked whether my donor's name was Tim L., there was a momentary pause.

"No, no, you can't know that," Gail finally said. "I'm not supposed to discuss this with you. Please, Claire, let it go. Even if you succeed in tracking down the family, you'd just be opening a can of worms."

"What do you mean?"

"You can never predict how the donor's family will respond. People in these situations have all kinds of unexpected reactions. If you're curious about the donor, I don't blame you; I'd be curious too. But please let it go. This whole topic is too emotional and too volatile."

I was disappointed by Gail's response, and a little surprised. But I respected her judgment and I assured her that I would drop the subject.

But the subject refused to drop me.

I would gradually learn a lot more about my donor. And eventually I would discover that my amazing dream about Tim L. was more true than I ever imagined.

Two

First Position

I GREW UP with a different sense of self than the one I live with now. As a very young child I was part of an extended family that was close and mostly happy. My father was a physician, and during World War II, when he was overseas with the army, we three — my mother, my older sister, Marilyn, and I — lived with my mother's parents in the Bronx.

My grandparents were poor and their apartment was tiny, and had they not been so welcoming it would have seemed cramped. My mother, grandmother, and I shared a bed, sleeping head to toe. Marilyn slept on a cot, and my grandfather spent his nights on the living room couch. It was a warm and traditional Jewish household, rich in food and good humor, where we celebrated the Sabbath with Friday night dinners at a table crowded with relatives. Although these memories now seem to have emanated from some other lifetime, they still resonate with stability, engagement, and pure emotional comfort.

My grandparents, Chana and Sholom, had not always enjoyed such a peaceful life. In 1913 they had escaped from Czarist Russia with my mother, who was then three years old; two boys, my uncles Hy and Lou, were born later, in New York. Although my grandparents rarely spoke of their former lives, I knew they had survived several pogroms, and that my grandmother had evaded one particularly vicious rampage by hiding in a barrel. As a girl I retained a vivid mental image of these two adults and their small child being pursued by bloodthirsty Cossacks on horses, literally running to the boat that would carry them to America. Perhaps it didn't happen exactly that way, but even today, the memory of my grandparents still brings to mind a series of dangerous episodes and narrow escapes.

Although my grandparents had been exposed to much sorrow and suffering, they were kind, compassionate, and incredibly optimistic. "Money they couldn't give me," my uncle Lou said years later, "but they were loaded with hope." Grandma was always reminding us that today's troubles would pass soon enough, and that, in a phrase she must have uttered a thousand times, "tomorrow will be better."

She was a tiny woman, while Grandpa, who worked as a paperhanger, was a big, bald man who sparkled and glistened and looked like a Jewish Mister Clean. He had a great sense of humor, especially about his financial struggles. "You know, Claire," he would say with his heavy Yiddish accent, "I'm actually very successful. I came to this country with every intention of being a poor man, and you'll notice that I achieved my goal."

Unlike many couples of their generation, my grandparents were not only life partners, but true friends as well. They had long talks in Yiddish, and while they spoke English to their grandchildren, both my grandparents and parents reverted to Yiddish when the topic was deemed inappropriate for younger ears. Naturally, with such a powerful incentive, Marilyn and I learned a lot of Yiddish phrases.

In my grandparents' home, dreams were a natural and recurring topic of discussion. This was common among Russian Jewish immigrants: if you had a dream during the night, you talked about it in the morning. The adults would offer each other interpretations, but there was no psychological component to these conversations. There were recognized symbols: if you dreamed X, it meant Y. There's an adage in the Talmud that an uninterpreted dream is like an unopened letter; in our family, you might say, we always read our mail.

When it came to dreams, everyone deferred to my grandmother. We thought of her as a bit of a gypsy, because in addition to her fondness for dreams, she would occasionally foretell the future with a deck of cards. Some of her dreams, too, pointed to future events or possibilities, but others were mundane and even practical. If a number appeared to her in the night, she would go down to the candy store the next day to play that number with a two-cent or a nickel bet. She sometimes dreamed about her childhood in Russia, but on that painful topic she was mostly silent.

Even her health was bound up with dreams. Grandma almost died in the flu epidemic of 1918, and she was so weak that my mother and her brother Hy, who were eight and five, had to spend a year in a loveless and rat-infested orphanage. When she recovered, Grandma dreamed about a mysterious, bearded stranger who held a staff over her head and promised that from that day on she would never again know sickness. "Never" is a long time, but for the next fifteen years she was the picture of health.

Growing up, I learned to pay attention to my own dreams, and to regard them, at least some of the time, as either true or potentially true. This applied not only to night dreams, but also to daydreams, hopes, wishes, and all other expressions of imagination and desire. If a dream wasn't literally true when you dreamed it, you could always work very hard to try to make it true. I learned to see dreams as a powerful motivating force that can propel you to overcome enormous obstacles. Of course, as my grandmother would have added, it also doesn't hurt to be lucky.

I wasn't exactly lucky, but I did have a number of experiences that might be called psychic. When a woman in our neighborhood became pregnant, I knew about it before she told anyone. I don't know how or why; I just *knew*. When an item was lost, I could often find it. When I went roller skating with my friends, one popular contest rewarded those skaters who ended up in a particular corner of the rink when the music stopped; I often knew which corner it would be, and even when the music would stop. These things happen to most people every now and then; they seemed to happen to me a lot.

Long before I ever heard of Jung, or his idea of synchronicity, I had concluded that coincidences aren't necessarily random, and that "accidents" sometimes happen by design. Events often unfold for a reason, even when that reason isn't necessarily clear. Mysterious forces are at work in the universe that affect our lives in ways we don't always understand.

During my childhood, I often had the sense of knowing things that weren't necessarily clear to other people, although I assumed they were. I was uncomfortable, for example, when anyone in our family or our neighborhood made a disparaging remark about other ethnic or religious groups. It wasn't only the bigotry that upset me; I was genuinely baffled by these comments. As a child, it was clear to me not only that everyone belonged to the same human family, but that each of us contained parts and elements of other people. I also knew that we had all been alive in previous incarnations. I was sure, for example, that my mother had been a Catholic not so long ago — and perhaps even a Catholic who disliked Jews. This view of the world was so self-evident to me that I couldn't believe it wasn't known to everyone. But while children are especially open and receptive to such ideas, as they get older they conform to an adult society whose organizing principles, at least these days, leave little room for metaphysical reflections.

Like my grandmother, I've had powerful and unusual dreams all my life, and decades later, one dream in particular still haunts me. A few weeks after Ira, my first husband, and I were married, Ira's father died. Artie's body was cremated, and after the funeral we all gathered at his house in Westchester. The ashes were in the car, and Ira and his brothers planned to scatter them the following day in one of their father's favorite places. Exhausted after the funeral, I went to sleep early in Ira's old room with the moonlight shining through the window. Then I had the dream.

> *The doorbell rings, and when I run downstairs to answer it, I see the spirit of Artie. I am terrified, because I know that Artie's spirit has returned to select someone who will go with him. Although I'm not sure what this means, the prospect of going with Artie to this unknown place fills me with dread.*
>
> *Now I am outside the house. As I watch, Ira's two brothers jump out the window and disappear. Then the front door opens and Ira comes out; he begins walking away, and I follow him.*

I awoke from this dream literally trembling with fear, because I thought Ira and I were supposed to die. Just then, Ira came bounding into the room. Before I could speak, he said, "I don't want to wait until tomorrow. I've got to scatter the ashes right now."

"All right," I said, "I'll go with you. Let me put some clothes on and we'll get them from the car."

"The ashes aren't in the car," he said. "I brought them up and put them right here, under the bed."

Holy Moses! When I heard that, I couldn't believe it.

Ira and I left the house with Artie's ashes and started walking. So *that's* what the dream meant, I thought. We really *were* supposed to go with Artie, but that didn't mean we had to die. As we scattered his ashes, I began to breathe easier. But what an amazing dream.

I concluded that Artie's spirit had contacted me with a message, and that Ira had obviously received a similar message at exactly the same time, through some other channel. Dreams are a common transmitting device, but there are surely others, even if we don't have names for them.

Sadly, the years of warmth and security in my grandparents' apartment came to an early end. In 1945, when I was five, my father returned from the war and the four of us moved into our own place. But we missed the stabilizing, loving presence of our grandparents, and without them the family dynamics were very different.

My mother was a troubled woman, who was often unpredictable and sometimes mean. Living with her produced so much anxiety that I sometimes wondered how the only daughter of my affectionate, dependable grandparents could have turned out as she did. She was often cranky and jealous, and she'd lash out at the slightest provocation — mostly at my sister, who, as the older child, bore the brunt of these seemingly arbitrary eruptions.

I don't have a good explanation for my mother's instability. It's possible that one of its causes was a terrible frustration from never having realized her dream of devoting her life to some artistic pursuit. She played the piano, and she spoke with pride about having acted in plays during high school. Later, when I became a dancer, the intensity of her support and her devoted attention to my career sometimes made me wonder if she wasn't living vicariously through me.

In my adult life my mother and I were finally able to be friends, and later on, when she was dying, she wanted me at her side. Mother, I thought, you brought me into this world and I'm here to see you out. As I prayed for her on her deathbed, I also prayed for myself — that I would be able to let go of those negative qualities in her that also belonged to me.

As a child I often prayed for a different mother — a warm and tender woman who was more like the mothers of my girlfriends. These mothers, or so I imagined, were close to their daughters and openly loving, and would never dream of yelling at them for no good reason. I yearned for the closeness and warmth I had felt with my grandparents, and I longed for the unconditional love that my mother seemed unable to provide.

At the same time, I also admired her. She had studied hard to escape her impoverished childhood, and although her own mother could neither read nor write, my mother went to college and became a high school English teacher. She was bright and capable, with flashes of kindness and generosity. She had excellent taste, and loved antiques and beautiful things. She had many friends and loved to throw parties, where she was a beautiful and gracious hostess. And, like her father, she had a terrific sense of humor.

Like many troubled individuals, my mother had a way of cutting straight to the heart of the matter. She was full of insight, and although she often muddied up an issue with her negativity, she generally spoke the truth. I have no doubt that she loved

Marilyn and me, but sadly for all three of us, she found it far easier to display anger than affection.

My father, fortunately, provided some balance; he was consistent, caring, and supportive. Although he constantly tried to appease my mother, he wasn't strong enough to stand up to her, and was never able to get her the help she obviously needed. Marilyn and I appreciated his kindness, but even that led to problems when my mother became jealous of his relatively uncomplicated relationship with us.

What made life bearable was our small summer cottage on Swan Lake in the Catskills, where we spent every summer together with our grandparents. Dad was the town doctor, and more than one family dinner was interrupted when some unlucky fisherman came by with a hook embedded in his hand. Cousins were always dropping in to share meals at our oval red Formica table with the matching red bench, and for a few weeks each year we were able to return to happier times. Even my mother was relatively relaxed at Swan Lake, but because of a fight she'd had with our next-door neighbors, Marilyn and I weren't allowed to play with their kids. But everything is relative, and Swan Lake was far better than home. I loved that place, and I continued going there until well into my twenties. My parents eventually sold it, but to this day I still return there in my dreams.

I responded to my mother's volatility by tuning out. At dinner I would sit there quietly, waiting for the inevitable eruption. The moment the yelling began I would mentally pull down a curtain and wall myself off, creating a private, secret space that my mother's anger could not penetrate. Later, in college, what I appreciated most of all were the daily meals in the cafeteria. It wasn't the food, but the surprising revelation that dinner could be both pleasant and predictable.

When things became noisy at home, I would imagine myself as part of some other household. I thought constantly about growing up and getting out, as far as possible from all of this abuse and conflict. At home or in public, my mother was always on the attack, humiliating my sister and me in front of our friends. When I was a teenager, my boyfriends were afraid to come to the house to take me out.

I followed my own path and became a closet rebel. I smiled and said yes to everything, but I did as I pleased. With Marilyn as the lightning rod for my mother's anger, I generally got off easy. My sister covered for me, and sometimes she even took the blame for my mischief.

When I was a young adult, living on my own, I called my mother to tell her I was getting married. Nobody in the family had met Ira, and I heard later that my mother told her friends that she wasn't even sure whether Claire's future husband was white. The fact that my mother actually wondered about this says a lot about how she perceived me. Although interracial marriages were extremely rare in those days, she thought of me as being capable of such a socially daring and rebellious act. Ira was white, but my mother's assessment of me was accurate.

Children who are unhappy at home sometimes find redemption at school, but I didn't. I couldn't master a subject unless I saw its relevance or at least found it interesting. Because Marilyn excelled at school, the two of us soon became pegged as the smart one and the pretty one. It took years before I finally realized that I, too, had brains, and that Marilyn was good-looking. Until then, my self-esteem was pretty low.

I also found it hard to make the standard, logical connections that seemed to come naturally to my classmates. This may have been a response to the emotional instability of our home, but every year, for example, the Christmas school vacation came as a total surprise. I didn't expect it, and I couldn't seem to grasp the idea that certain events occurred at regular, predictable points in the annual cycle. There wasn't a rounded continuity to my life.

But what really set me apart were my health problems. At the age of three I was diagnosed with a congenital heart murmur that I expected to live with all my life. "Whatever Claire does," the doctor warned my parents, "don't let it get too strenuous." Although I was an active child, my parents worried about my health and treated me as if I were frail. I certainly didn't feel frail, although I suffered from low blood sugar. At my father's suggestion, I always carried some candy with me in case I suffered a disorienting attack. My condition was a forerunner to diabetes, which ran in our family.

I also had trouble breathing on hot, humid days. My body would become dehydrated, and I could practically feel myself losing weight. Shortly after Ira and I were married, we traveled in Africa, where I almost died in Dakar. It looked like a case of malaria, but what really did me in was the incredible humidity.

As a child I came down with a great many colds and sore throats, which usually developed into bronchitis or the flu. While I didn't see myself as sickly, I didn't feel entirely healthy, either. And even when I felt fine, I was always aware of a serious imperfection at the center of my being.

Because of my heart, I wasn't allowed to enter races or participate in any rigorous activities. Marilyn was given the difficult job of looking out for me — an assignment that placed an enormous and unfair burden on her because I was often rambunctious and uncooperative.

Although Marilyn knew that my heart murmur was real, she always suspected that my many lesser ailments might be caused by a desire for more attention. I hated these insinuations, but I now believe that my sister was at least partly right. While I wasn't faking, I definitely experienced some secondary gains from being sick. I was happy to miss school, but a more important consideration was that my normally unpredictable mother became loving and attentive during my illnesses, and would bring me baked potatoes with butter and sour cream. (Years later I would do the same for my own daughter.) Even after I was married, whenever I was sick my mother would either come to see me or she'd send my father.

During this mostly unhappy childhood, dance was my salvation, my rescuer, my antidote to depression. I started dancing at the age of eight, and as soon as I had found my calling, I fell under its spell forever. I believed I was born to dance, and I can still remember sitting on the radiator in my bedroom and looking out the window at the night sky: I found a star and made a wish that I would become a great ballerina. I also promised myself that one way or another, dance would always be part of my life. And it has been — through several decades, in sickness and in health.

Throughout my childhood and adolescence, in high school and college, dance was a way out of my misery, a powerful and spiritual alternative to our contentious family life. No matter what was happening at home, I could leave it behind the moment the music started. Some dancers feel they become another person when they dance, but I felt I was expressing the best parts of myself — the *real* me, the creative me, the person I was meant to become. I often became lost in the music, although it might be more accurate to say that I was lost *before* the music, and that dancing was more like being found.

When I was ten, the dance teacher at summer camp selected me for the lead role in *Snow White,* whereupon I announced to my parents that I was going to become a ballerina. Impossible, they said. A girl with a heart problem can't be a dancer! But I was already hooked, and their anxieties about my health only strengthened my resolve. Dance now took on the additional glow of forbidden fruit and became part of my rebellion. Finally, after I begged and pleaded, they allowed me to take ballet lessons on Saturdays. One class led to another, and it soon became clear that I had a passion, possibly even a gift.

When I was eleven, my ballet teacher took me to see a performance of *Giselle*, which epitomizes romantic ballet. *Giselle* is the story of a young girl who is determined to dance, but whose mother tries to prevent her from realizing her dream because of Giselle's weak heart.

At least that's what I thought *Giselle* was about. Later, when I saw it again as an adult, I realized that for decades I had been carrying around a distorted version of the story, and that Giselle's heart problem is one minor detail in a long and elaborate story. Seeing *Giselle* as a young girl's struggle to dance in spite of her heart condition is a little like viewing *Hamlet* as the story of a young man who kills his girlfriend's loquacious father: it's factual, but not really true. I obviously needed to see *Giselle* as the playing out of my own struggle.

A few months later, my parents took me to a movie that reinforced the dramatic impact of *Giselle*. *Limelight,* one of Charlie Chaplin's last films, portrays an unlikely romance between an aging clown (Chaplin) and a beautiful young ballerina (Claire Bloom). As the film opens, the dancer has just tried to kill herself. What drove her to such despair? She'd had a serious illness that prevented her from dancing! *Limelight* is an enormously affecting movie, and when it was over I burst into tears. To this day I can't watch it without crying.

Although I didn't consciously realize this at the time, *Giselle* and *Limelight* were variations on the same theme: the near-death and subsequent resurrection of a young, dark-haired dancer. I took this idea to heart, and saw it as *my* story and *my* destiny. As things turned out, it really *was* my story, although at the time I couldn't begin to imagine that years later, after nearly dying, I would almost literally be resurrected into a new life in which I really would dance again. Throughout my youth, I assumed that my heart murmur was the biggest obstacle I would ever have to face. Little did I know!

As I continued taking dance classes with no detrimental effects on my health, my parents became more flexible. They were proud of my successes, and over time their apprehensions about my heart began to fade. I did my part by always restraining myself a little and holding back. I was grateful to be dancing at all, and I didn't want to risk any further damage to my heart.

As a teenager I faced another barrier when I quickly shot up to my current height of five feet, six inches. This wouldn't be a problem today, but during the 1950s I was considered slightly too tall for ballet. I was shattered, but when one of my friends suggested that I look into modern dance, I took her advice. To my surprise, I soon came to love this completely different style of dance, which struck me as less constrained, more expressive, and more emotionally satisfying than ballet. And while I have always appreciated classical dance, I soon realized that for me, with my artistic drive and rebellious spirit, modern was a better choice.

In high school I took classes at Juilliard with Pearl Lang, a disciple of Martha Graham, who invited me to join her company for a Hanukkah festival performance at Madison Square Garden. I could hardly believe I was working with real dancers in a professional company! I even received a modest check, which meant that I, too, could now consider myself a professional.

I pushed ahead and won a scholarship, which I used for a summer program at the Connecticut College for Women. Here I was fortunate enough to study with some of the leading figures in modern dance, including José Limón, Lucas Hoving, and Alwin Nikolais. I even took a class with Martha Graham, and one memorable morning she slapped my hip into proper position while demonstrating a contraction. This was a big deal: Martha Graham was regarded as a deity, and it was considered a great honor to be touched by her.

After high school I was accepted at Adelphi College (now Adelphi University) on Long Island, one of the few schools to offer a dance major in the 1950s. Adelphi was close enough to Manhattan that students could easily attend Broadway shows, dance classes, and auditions. My first audition, an open call for the film version of *West Side Story,* was conducted by Jerome Robbins himself. Hundreds of dancers tried out for two places, and Mr. Robbins had me dancing all day. Finally, when only four of us were left, he politely sent me home.

I was crushed not to be chosen after coming so close, but on the train back to school I was able to take a longer view. Don't feel too badly, I told myself. You did great, and this was just your first audition. There will be many others.

But there weren't. In the spring of my senior year, my feet suddenly swelled up for no apparent reason. I was diagnosed with glomerulonephritis, a kidney disease. Although I felt no pain, I had to spend a month at Mt. Sinai Hospital, leaving only to attend my senior prom and graduation. When I was released, the doctor took me aside and gave me the terrible news: I could never dance again. And in case that wasn't awful enough, it would be dangerous for me to have children.

I was devastated. A few weeks later, when I looked up glomerulonephritis in a medical book, I was shocked to see that people often died from it. My parents, who had finally over-come their fears about my heart murmur, now insisted that I move back home after graduation so they could take care of me. But I wouldn't hear of it. Now that my life was pretty much ruined, the last thing I wanted was to return home. Instead, I rented an apartment with a friend on Manhattan's Upper West Side and reassured my parents that I wouldn't dance.

It was terribly hard, but I really did stop. Giving up my dream was excruciating, but for all my rebelliousness, in those days I still believed doctors were God-like. It didn't even occur to me to challenge their wisdom.

Not dancing was enormously painful for me, and I soon found that watching other dancers was just as bad. I remem-bered clearly what every step and motion felt like, and to see these movements being performed without being able to do them myself was more than I could endure. Like a recovering alcoholic, I found it better to separate myself entirely from my previous pleasure: I stopped going to dance events and avoided any music that reminded me of dancing. My life's dream had dis-solved, and everything I had wished for was over.

What new self had I become, now that my body and spirit were no longer dancing? I wasn't sure, except that this new me had no discipline, no goal, no calling, no plan, no dream. I lived for the moment: I drank, I smoked, and I ate without limits. By the standards of a dancer, I soon became fat and out of shape. For years my body had defined my dream and put it into prac-tice; I didn't realize that my purest essence, the part of me that had been expressed through dance, would always be there. When I stopped dancing, I thought it was gone forever.

For all my disappointment, however, I didn't succumb to despair or give up on life. I was determined to find my own way, whatever that turned out to be, and I loved being on my own and living in Manhattan. Although I quickly lost touch with most of my college friends, who had all been dancers, I made new friends who worked in business, advertising, or the theater.

I drifted in and out of several jobs, including a secretarial position and a stint as a hostess in a restaurant. Because I had studied English in college, I was able to find a job in publishing — sort of. Okay, so *Hairdo Magazine* wasn't exactly Alfred A. Knopf, but sometimes even the wrong job can lead to good things. One day a new girl showed up in the office, a music and dance enthusiast whose boyfriend was a musician with the Alvin Ailey Dance Company. Maureen Meloy lived a block from me, and when I told her about my previous life, she encouraged me to join a gym and start working out, and didn't let up on me until I did. Soon she was pushing copies of *Variety* under my nose and urging me to start dancing again.

"But I *can't*," I explained for the umpteenth time. "I was sick, remember?"

"That was then," she said. "Maybe things have changed." She handed me a notice and said, "Read this."

Helen Tamiris and Daniel Nagrin, two well-known names in the small world of modern dance, were seeking another member for their company. Although I was busy on the day of the audition, Maureen insisted that I call to ask if they would see me at another time.

How brazen, I thought, but Maureen was so convincing that I called. To my amazement, Tamiris and Nagrin scheduled a private audition in their apartment and studio on West 72nd Street. Nervous, overweight, and still smoking, I danced for them and gave them my résumé. Fortunately, the audition included plenty of improvisation, which was always my strength. Even so, I left the studio with few expectations. "We'll be in touch," I was told. Sure, I thought.

Two weeks later, when I had all but given up, Daniel Nagrin called and offered me the job. I couldn't believe it! The next morning I went into work and gave Maureen an enormous hug. We soon lost touch, but I still wonder about this woman who appeared out of nowhere and completely changed my life. Actually, Maureen was one of several people who seem to have been sent to me over the years, as if by some higher power, to move my life along in an important new direction. I don't pretend to understand this mysterious phenomenon, except that I know it happens to some people, and I'm profoundly grateful that it happened to me.

I promptly quit my job at *Hairdo* and began a six-week training program as the eighth and newest member of the Tamiris-Nagrin company. "We were right to hire you," Daniel Nagrin told me after two weeks. "Soon we'll be giving you solos. I'm amazed at how quickly you've stopped smoking, lost weight, and improved your skills."

It wasn't amazing to me; all I needed was the incentive. I was dedicated and devoted to dance, and when this incredible opportunity opened up, I rushed to embrace it.

Before the training program began, I had checked in with my kidney doctor at Mt. Sinai. With this opportunity in my life, I probably would have resumed dancing in any case, no matter what the risks. But to my astonishment, the doctor told me that my kidneys had healed, and that after four years I could finally stop taking the medications. I could dance!

"This is really incredible," he said. "I wish I could tell you why you got better, but I have no idea." He showed me the medical records of another patient, a young boy who had come to the hospital with glomerulonephritis around the same time I had. "Look at this," he said. "Your numbers are identical, and you both had the same prognosis. But today you're dancing, this poor kid is dying, and I can't explain why."

I couldn't either. It certainly wasn't the medications, which were never intended as a cure. All I know is that these things happen, and that physical healing sometimes takes place in a realm far removed from the treatments and cures of conventional medicine. Perhaps, in this case, my body cured itself. But why? It could have been my strong will to live, although the boy who was dying may have had an equally strong will. Perhaps I got better because it just wasn't my time to die, and God had something else in mind for me. I simply don't know the answer.

I went on to dance, first with Tamiris and Nagrin, and then with Gloria Contraras in her ballet company. I spent a year with Gloria in Mexico, and then returned to America, where I performed with several companies and taught dance at various schools and colleges. I married Ira, and although the kidney doctor had warned me that getting pregnant could be very dangerous, I decided to take the risk. I wanted to be a mother as much as I wanted to dance. After a wonderful pregnancy, my two great loves came together: Amara was born in 1972, and before she could even walk we were already dancing together.

Three

Bad News

FOR SEVERAL YEARS, until I married Ira, I performed with various modern dance companies and taught dance at Hunter College High School and Barnard College. Shortly after our wedding, I gave it all up when Ira and I decided to travel through Europe and Africa. We ended up living in Spain for a year, where I studied flamenco dance and Ira, a photographer, worked on his portfolio.

After two years abroad, we returned to New York and settled down to begin a family. Just before Amara was born, we moved to a house overlooking the ocean in Hull, Massachusetts, on Boston's south shore. By then, however, our marriage was coming apart, and two years later, we divorced. Ira remained an attentive father, and we became friends in a way that hadn't seemed possible while we were married.

A year after my divorce a new man came into my life. David and I were together for ten years, including three years of marriage. During this period I set up our local arts council, opened a dance school, and performed in several regional productions. Unfortunately this marriage, too, came to an end. Apparently I wasn't very good at marriage, but while I became shy about matrimony, I didn't give up on romance.

Which brings me to the spring of 1985, when I was forty-five and my life was going well. I was in love again — would I never learn? — and was finishing my first year as a drama teacher at Brookline High, a wonderful school near Boston where the students were eager to learn. Amara and I were now living in Brookline, where I rented an apartment. But I still owned the house in Hull, which we used on weekends and in the summer.

Over breakfast on a pleasant Sunday morning, I picked up *Parade* magazine, which comes with the Sunday *Boston Globe*. Cher was on the cover. Flipping through it, I noticed an attractive, smiling woman who looked to be roughly my age. Her name was Mary Gohlke, and I read that four years earlier she had been the first person to survive a combined heart-lung transplant. I couldn't imagine it, so I started reading her story, which began when she had started feeling tired and short of breath for no apparent reason. After running some tests, her doctor said, "You have a very serious disease called primary pulmonary hypertension."

When I read those words I nearly fell off my chair. Eighteen months earlier I had been given the very same diagnosis by my own doctor, who had definitely *not* used the phrase "very serious disease." I had gone to see him after feeling tired on the dance floor and slightly winded when I climbed stairs. At first I had ignored these symptoms. It's middle age, I told myself. You're out of shape. Get some exercise. Lose a few pounds.

But at a deeper level I was concerned. Why was I suddenly so tired when I had been dancing for years, through countless grueling rehearsals, exhausting classes, and strenuous performances? Just a few years earlier, at the relatively old age of thirty-nine, I had performed the demanding lead dance role in a local production of *Oklahoma!* But now, for some reason, I was always out of breath.

Dr. Sage, my cardiologist, found that the right side of my heart was enlarged. After further tests, he said I had primary pulmonary hypertension. He didn't elaborate, and at the time — although it seems inconceivable to me now — I didn't ask. But if he had used the word "serious," or even "disease," I would have remembered.

"The good news is that you won't be needing surgery," he had said. "We can control this problem through medication."

Although the medication didn't help much, I thought of myself as having a condition rather than an illness. Incredibly, it hadn't occurred to me to do any research about primary pulmonary hypertension (PPH) — or even to look it up in a medical book. But now, in *Parade* magazine, I read that PPH closes the blood vessels in the lungs, which in turn forces the heart to work harder.

As I read on, I learned something else that hit me like a gigantic hammer: PPH was more than a serious disease. It was terminal.

Oh my God.

I said nothing to Amara. She was thirteen, which was certainly old enough to understand my anxiety. But why alarm her now? Maybe I was jumping to conclusions. But when I went to see Dr. Sage, he confirmed that what I had read about PPH was correct. He explained that the word "primary" meant that this disease had no known cause; it also had no known cure. The reason he hadn't told me these things before, he said, was that he hadn't wanted to alarm me. Besides, my case was fairly mild.

I asked Dr. Sage if I should be thinking about a heart-lung transplant. Although I felt a little foolish asking about such a drastic solution, I had no intention of dying in my forties. And from what little I had just learned about PPH, there didn't seem to be much middle ground between doing nothing and taking extreme measures. People say their priorities become clear during a crisis, and when I learned the truth about my illness, my priorities were so clear you could see through them. I wanted to live, and I wanted Amara to continue to have a mother.

"Fortunately," the doctor said, "you're still in good health. Later on, if things change, I suppose a transplant might be your ace in the hole."

It gave me a shiver to hear this cautious, measured man acknowledge that such a terrifying procedure might someday become necessary. This was crazy! A week ago I didn't even know I was sick, and now, suddenly, I was talking with my doctor about the possibility of receiving a new heart and lungs. It boggled the mind.

As our conversation drew to a close, something clicked in my brain. Although I was only dimly aware of it at the time, I know now that a fundamental change occurred in my consciousness that day. I realized that ignorance about PPH was doing me no good, and that Dr. Sage's feel-good approach was discouraging me from taking control of my health. I would continue to seek the advice of doctors, but this illness was my problem and my responsibility. I would start by learning everything I could about it.

Had Dr. Sage been wrong not to disclose the whole truth about my illness? Today, the question seems more complicated than I once believed. On one level, yes; he certainly should have told me the full story right away. At the same time, it's simplistic and a little too convenient to blame the doctor in this case. Physicians are influenced as much by their patients as by their training, and most patients would rather leave the important decisions to an omnipotent father figure.

I used to be one of those patients. Dr. Sage had shielded me from the truth not only with the best of intentions, but also because I, as the passive, acquiescent patient, had invited him to do so. Now, as I geared up to save my own life, I had to become less of a patient — less *patient*, you might say — and more of a consumer. I had been thrust into battle, and it was time to start fighting.

But that's easier said than done. For all my determination to learn about PPH, I found it enormously difficult to move ahead. I was frightened, and what little I knew about this disease was bad enough; I wasn't all that eager to learn more. Ignorance wasn't bliss, exactly, but as a first cousin to denial, it seemed to offer a little comfort. Maybe the bad news could wait a little longer.

But when I saw myself backsliding, I pushed forward. Fear is understandable, I told myself, but I can't give in to it. I have to push through the fear. Establish some control. I have a terrible disease, and before I can figure out what to do, I need as much information as possible. This isn't cancer or heart disease, I realized, where a patient can afford to close her eyes a little because the doctors have plenty of experience with these problems. PPH was so rare that most doctors knew nothing about it. My internist had never even seen a patient who had it, and I soon learned why: this disease strikes one person in a million. No wonder my internist referred me to a pulmonary specialist.

I kept hoping the specialist would tell me that Dr. Sage had made an honest mistake, and that I had something that looked a lot like PPH but was far less serious. But the specialist confirmed the diagnosis and recommended that I take an aspirin a day as a blood thinner. This was really depressing, and it seemed to symbolize the pathetic weakness of my arsenal. Here I was with a fatal disease, and the best I could do was to take one lousy *aspirin*?

I called the National Institutes of Health in Bethesda and asked for everything they had about PPH. I also bought a copy of Mary Gohlke's book, *I'll Take Tomorrow*. As I feared, it provided a far more harrowing account of PPH than the brief and relatively sanitized excerpt I had read in *Parade*. More than once, I noticed that my hand was trembling as I turned the page. How could I ever cope with all the physical and emotional problems that Mary described in such frightening and vivid detail?

The breathing problems were bad enough, but it was the emotional pain that really got to me. I was crying as I read how Mary's husband had reached across the breakfast table, taken her hand, and gently asked where she wanted to be buried. Or when she tearfully explained to her teenage son that she was dying. Would I soon need to have a similar conversation with Amara? So far I hadn't said much about my illness, and she hadn't asked. But sooner or later I'd have to tell her. Where would I find the strength?

To some extent, I had already found it. Although parts of Mary's book were frightening, I was inspired by her courage, and by how she took charge of her own diminishing life. Her doctors had tried to discourage her from seeking the transplant because the operation was experimental and dangerous. And it was both, no question about it. But Mary had decided that a risky operation was still better than a slow and painful death, and I felt the same way.

Now, at least, I had a role model, a pioneer who had been through this illness and had survived. As long as Mary Gohlke was alive, PPH no longer had a perfect record. Now there was a precedent, and a reason to hope.

When I finished the book I actually called the author on the phone. I had never done this before, but Mary lived in Phoenix, her number was listed, and I dialed it. It was hard to believe, but moments after reading a book that had already changed my life, I was speaking to the author.

Or *not* speaking, to be precise, because when she said "Hello?" and I said, "Mary Gohlke?" and she said, "Yes" — that's all it took: I burst into tears. I tried to explain why I was calling, which was difficult because I didn't really *know* why. I just wanted to hear her voice, which would mean she was still alive, which would mean that maybe I, too, could survive.

"It's all right," she said. "I wrote the book for you, and for others who are going through this frightening and lonely time. I'll give you some advice. Be positive, because an optimistic attitude can help your immune system. Set a goal for each day — even if there are days when your goal is nothing more than staying alive until tomorrow. Find the strength to keep going, and never give up."

I listened carefully, knowing that I might soon be needing this advice. Meanwhile, I studied the information that arrived from Bethesda — every grim word of it. The bottom line, as I already knew, was that PPH is incurable. It weakens the muscles in the pulmonary artery and its branches until high blood pressure in the lungs leads to failure in the right side of the heart. I also learned that PPH is often difficult to diagnose, which meant, I imagined, that things could have been even worse. For whatever it might be worth, Dr. Sage had detected it early.

According to the literature, the progression of PPH differed for each person. Dr. Sage had mentioned this, but he had neglected to tell me that even so, almost everybody with PPH had one thing in common. Within three to five years, they were dead.

Over the next few weeks, my symptoms grew noticeably worse. As the summer heat grew stronger, the tiredness I had been feeling during the school year became more intense. On bad days, when I woke up in the morning it took all my energy just to wash my face and brush my teeth. Then, exhausted, I'd have to return to bed.

Amara was away at camp, but I was grateful for my boyfriend, Alan, who was taking good care of me. Alan looked in on me often. I could see how difficult it was becoming for him to watch me turn into a pale shadow of the vigorous, energetic woman he had known for several years. As August began, my body became harder and harder to lug around. What about my teaching, which was scheduled to resume after Labor Day? This was the best job I'd ever had, and I couldn't wait for the school year to begin. But would I be strong enough to go back?

I wasn't. The school administration was wonderful: they assured me that the job was mine whenever I was well enough to return, and they even paid me my salary. I was astonished and grateful to be treated so well after only one year on the job.

When I looked back on the previous year, it was hard to believe how thoroughly I had ignored and denied the true state of my health. Although I felt increasingly worn down as the months went by, I pretended that nothing was wrong. In the spring, when I climbed the stairs on my way to the cafeteria, I often felt that I was turning into a younger version of my grandmother at the end of her life. "'S'no good, 's'no good," she would tell me as she slowly made her way up the rickety wooden stairs to her apartment, while I followed close behind, helping her schlep those heavy bundles of groceries. She seemed so old, this frail little woman whom I loved so much, and now, finally, I understood. I was only in my forties, but I understood. 'S'no good, Grandma. 'S'no good.

I tried to mask my fatigue. I didn't want anyone to know how weak I was feeling, and that included me. When other teachers were around, I'd make excuses. "Go ahead," I'd tell them. "I'm looking for something." Then I'd rummage through my bag until my colleagues were out of sight.

During the fall semester I had sat on the floor to lead the students in their warm-up exercises, but by the spring I couldn't even open or close the windows. We were preparing a production of *Pippin,* and my codirector told me later that he thought I was slacking off and acting like a princess.

One day at rehearsal I was watching a dance scene I had choreographed when I noticed a step that looked wrong. I was so focused on the play that I forgot my limitations and bounded up the three steps to the stage. As I stood there panting and feeling as if I were about to collapse, the students became concerned. "Claire, are you all right?"

"Yeah, sure, just give me a minute."

Still, nobody knew. When the school day was over, I drove home and collapsed on my bed. Amara was out playing basketball, and a few minutes later she bounced into the apartment all flushed with fresh air and youth. I remember feeling painfully aware of the contrast between my daughter, in the flush of life, and my own, prematurely old body.

Sometimes I was jealous of the students and teachers around me, who seemed to be flying up the stairs. But I continued to guard my secret because working in this school was exciting and inspirational. I was teaching a new, experimental course on how to relieve stress through meditation and other techniques. My plan was to introduce the kinds of practical, real-life lessons I wished I could have learned in my own high school, and the kids were responding with enormous enthusiasm. It made sense that students in a high-powered, ambitious high school would welcome opportunities and techniques to reduce stress, and they seemed delighted to learn about stretching, yoga, meditation, and other ways of clearing their minds.

In September, I called Dr. Sage to report that my symptoms had become worse. He told me to come in for more tests, including a heart catheterization, an unpleasant procedure in which a tiny tube is threaded through one of your veins and is then pushed through all the way to your heart. Because you're given a local anesthetic, it's usually not painful. But for me it's always a creepy feeling when that catheter snakes its way through my body; it makes me feel terribly vulnerable. Unfortunately, there is no other way to take a precise reading of the blood pressures in the right side of the heart and the pulmonary artery.

I'd had this procedure done once before, back when Dr. Sage first determined that I had PPH. Now, as I gloomily looked ahead to my second catheterization, I remembered what I had learned from Dr. Herbert Benson, who had helped me through the first one. When I had told him how frightened I was, he encouraged me to make a mental effort to separate myself from the procedure. "You can actually watch it on a monitor," he told me. "While they're doing the catheterization, try to imagine yourself on another plane, looking down on the scene from above and thinking, *isn't this interesting.*" I tried it, and it definitely helped.

I had met Dr. Benson in 1974, when I developed high blood pressure after Ira and I were divorced. I was on medication, but I didn't like the idea of taking a powerful drug and staying on it for the rest of my life. There had to be a more natural way to solve this problem, although I couldn't quite imagine what that might be.

As it happened, Herb Benson had recently been written up in *The New York Times* for his innovative work in using relaxation techniques to treat physical disorders such as migraines, irregular heartbeats, and, especially, high blood pressure. I made an appointment, and during that initial visit, in the course of about ten minutes, Dr. Benson taught me how to meditate.

I don't mean to sound flip about this, because a ten-minute course in meditation might sound simplistic. But Benson had effectively taken the main ideas of Transcendental Meditation and reduced them to their essentials: Sit quietly in a regular place where you won't be disturbed. Close your eyes. Relax all your muscles, starting at your feet and progressing up to your head. Inhale through your nose, breathe out through your mouth, and on every outbreath silently say a special word or a brief prayer. (Benson suggested the word "one," which I still use.) Sit like that for twenty minutes. When distracting thoughts float by — and they invariably will — gently let them go and focus on your breathing.

There's a tendency to make meditation seem more difficult and mysterious than it really is, although for some people, I realize, it *is* difficult. I began meditating twice a day, and within a month my blood pressure had fallen so dramatically that I was able to cut my medication in half.*

Why did meditation work so well for me? First, I had a powerful incentive to succeed: my health depended on it. Second, as a dancer I'd had plenty of practice in maintaining focus and concentration, and in enlisting the powers of my mind to control my body. Finally, when Amara was born I had gone through natural childbirth, with its emphasis on concentrated, controlled breathing. I spent sixteen hours in labor, and next to that, believe me, a little meditation isn't all that difficult.

---

* I was one of many patients who lowered their blood pressure through meditation as part of a research project that became the basis of Dr. Benson's 1975 book, *The Relaxation Response*.

I have now been meditating every morning for over twenty years, and today I can't imagine life without it. In addition to helping me deal with stress, the clarity of mind that meditation produces often leads me to solve problems that have been weighing on me, even when I haven't been fully aware of them.

As I feared, the results of my second catheterization were grim: my pulmonary pressure had more than doubled. "Your illness is progressing rapidly," said Dr. Sage, "and I'm going to write to Johns Hopkins to ask if they'll see you for an evaluation."

"You mean for a transplant?"

"Yes."

I sighed. I knew that Hopkins was one of only three medical centers in the country that performed heart-lung transplants. If this optimist was thinking about a transplant, then I was really in trouble.

"Meanwhile, we'll put you on a blood thinner, and you'll probably be needing oxygen."

Which was his way of saying, *You're dying, and you don't have much time left.*

I had only one card left to play, and it looked like a long shot. Marilyn's husband, Mort, was a doctor in New York. He had been reading up on PPH, and he urged me to ask my doctor for a calcium channel blocker. It might not help, he admitted, but in some cases this medication can improve the heart's ability to pump blood. Dr. Sage was skeptical, but when I pressed him, he reluctantly wrote out a prescription for a drug called Procardia.

Now came the hardest part of all. I had to check out of the hospital, return home, and find some way to tell Amara I was dying. Because she had been away at camp most of the summer, she didn't really know how serious my condition was. Nothing could have prepared me for this agonizing moment, but I couldn't postpone it any longer.

Amara and I had always been close; even as a small child, she always had a part in whatever production I was choreographing at the time. But dance wasn't our only deep connection. Once, when she was younger, she ran into my room in the middle of the night to tell me about a particularly frightening dream. As she started talking, I started filling in details before she could say them. It was hard for either of us to believe, but we had both had the same dream at the same time.

And now we were about to share the same nightmare.

When I got home from the hospital I went straight to her bedroom. As we sat together on her white down comforter, I held Amara's hand and told her plainly what Dr. Sage had said. It was possible, I said, that I might qualify for a heart and lungs transplant, but that wasn't something we could count on. Even if I was accepted, the waiting list was very long because there were always more people who needed organs than there were donors.

When it comes to showing our emotions, Amara and I have always been very different. Even before my illness, she rarely wanted to talk about how she was feeling. When I told her what was going on, she kept her feelings to herself, and spent the next two days in her bedroom. I didn't actually see her crying, but her eyes were pink and puffy. I was crying for both of us — for Amara, who was too young to have to endure this terrible burden, and also for myself.

I had known for a while that I wasn't going to live to a ripe old age. But this latest news was devastating. More than anything, I wanted to hang on until Amara graduated. She had just started at Brookline High, although she hadn't much liked the idea of being in a school where her mother was teaching. We had laughed about this, and I had promised my daughter that I would go to great lengths to avoid embarrassing her in school. But now that was no longer an issue. Tomorrow I would call my supervisor and explain that I wasn't sure I would ever be healthy enough to return.

I felt so helpless. Please, God, don't let me die! And please protect Amara, who means more to me than my own life. Can you possibly keep me alive until she graduates?

Dr. Sage had promised to contact Johns Hopkins, and I hoped they would ask me to come down for an evaluation. But in my current condition it was hard to imagine even leaving the house, let alone flying to Baltimore. Dr. Sage had told me to arrange for regular deliveries of oxygen. I was also supposed to get a prescription filled for the blood thinner, and another one for the medication that Mort had recommended. But all of that would have to wait until the morning. Right now I was too exhausted and too depressed to even think about it.

Alan filled both prescriptions the next day, and I took my first dose of Procardia. I'm always leery of new medications, because I tend to react strongly to even a tiny dose. Although I imagined I had little to lose by trying Procardia, I was still frightened.

Half an hour after taking that first pill, I got up and sat in a chair, expecting to be gasping for breath. But nothing happened. I walked into the kitchen, again waiting for the inevitable shortness of breath. And again, nothing.

It was astounding! The change was so abrupt and so dramatic that I half feared I was dreaming. After taking the second pill, I stood by the window and looked down at the street. A young couple was walking together, and a boy ran past them. For the first time in months, I wasn't jealous. I watched the boy and I wasn't in awe of his youth.

This was real! I was starting to feel like a whole person again, like a child learning to walk. I didn't need the oxygen, and I didn't take the blood thinner. Over the next couple of weeks I regained most of my strength. I still had trouble climbing stairs, but nothing like before. Once again, I started going out in the world. And amazingly, I experienced no side effects.

But I also knew that I wasn't cured. Mort had warned me that even if the Procardia worked, it was only a temporary solution. At some point the drug would lose its efficacy. I understood that, but I was so grateful not to be actively dying that I almost didn't care.

Suddenly, I had a little breathing room — so to speak. The enemy had been driven back, at least for the moment, which allowed me to fortify myself against the next assault. I tried to be optimistic, but I was fully aware that my new miracle drug wouldn't last forever. And neither would I.

So now I had a few extra months, or maybe even a couple of years. Beyond that, who knew? My hope, of course, was that somebody would discover a cure for PPH. But I was also realistic. I didn't know what the future would bring, but I had a pretty good idea. Which is why I was so grateful for this unexpected reprieve, this gift of a little more time. The challenge was to use it wisely.

Four

Reprieve

THE FIRST THING I did was find a new doctor. Not only did I need a pulmonary specialist, but Dr. Sage was clearly too conservative for me. I told him so in a letter, in which I also described the extraordinary benefits I was receiving from Procardia. I refrained from adding that I was angry at him for his skepticism about the drug, and for not having informed me earlier that I had a serious and fatal disease. While he wasn't the right doctor for me, I genuinely liked the man and believed he had acted in good faith.

Changing doctors was a start, but I wanted to go further. What I was seeking, I now realized, was more than any physician could reasonably be expected to provide. I understood intuitively, if not yet intellectually, that the world of conventional medicine was simply too narrow for the questions and issues I was now facing. While I needed all the medical expertise I could find, I was also looking for somebody who could help me, both emotionally and spiritually, prepare for my own death.

One thing was clear: that person certainly wasn't the detached psychotherapist I had been seeing in recent months to deal with my mother's death and my second divorce. He had come highly recommended, and for a while he had been helpful, but only (and ironically) until I really needed him. When I told him I was dying, his response to this devastating news was swift, mechanical, and almost robotic. As always, he was sitting behind a huge desk that concealed most of his body and that now seemed to symbolize the considerable distance between us. "Oh, yes," he said when I told him the gloomy results and depressing implications of my recent tests. "Well, now, at this point you can expect to go through five distinct stages. In the first stage . . ."

Was he serious? I had just told him I was *dying,* and he wanted to recite the five stages of grief! No thanks; I could get that from a *book*! I had vaguely known that there wasn't much emotional connection between us, or a great deal of empathy emanating from him. But now it was painfully clear that he couldn't help me deal with my own mortality, the mother of all issues. I quickly ended the relationship.

For some time I had been hearing about a New Age therapist who specialized in treating clients with life-threatening illnesses, and who practiced his own blend of psychotherapy and spirituality. Rick Pisani, who had a medical degree and was trained as a conventional psychiatrist, had decided early in his career that he was more interested in holistic and alternative treatments. While I wasn't exactly sure what I was looking for, this man sounded promising, and I made an appointment to see him.

His office was on the second floor of a big old Victorian home. The house had plenty of warmth and character, with rich wood paneling on the walls and Oriental rugs on the floors. I had trouble getting up the long flight of stairs that led to his office, but when I made it to the top I immediately liked this warmhearted, kind-looking man with a trim beard, graying hair, and a most expressive face. And I noticed immediately that the chairs in his comfortable office faced each other, with no desk or table between them. I felt at home here, which made me optimistic about his ability to help me.

I quickly filled him in on the key events of my illness. "At some point during the next year or two," I said, "the medication will stop working. Unless I'm lucky enough to get a heart-lung transplant, I will be dying. I'm here because I'm looking for help in that process. I don't want to die, but if there's no choice, I'd like to prepare for death with a sense of equanimity. I meditate every day, but I need to go deeper. I'm also concerned about my daughter, and what will happen to her after I'm gone."

"That sounds reasonable," he said. "Let me tell you a little about what I do, and how I might be able to help. I work mostly with cancer patients, although a few clients have other terminal illnesses. My focus is on healing, but I want to be very clear as to how I'm using that word. I don't practice as a physician, so 'healing' doesn't refer to a cure, or a process where the patient's disease miraculously disappears. That happens on occasion, but it's rare and mysterious and you can't plan on it. As I use the word, a patient can be 'healed' during the illness and still die. In fact, some people are more healed and more whole when they're dying than at any other point in their lives. It's almost as if their physical weakness frees up a different kind of energy."

I nodded. While I appreciated what Dr. Pisani was saying, he struck me as being a little too comfortable with the inevitability of death. He might have been picking up on my reaction, for he added, "At the same time, I don't believe in closing the door or giving up. Bernie Siegel has a saying that I like: 'In the face of uncertainty, there's nothing wrong with hope.'"

"I understand," I said. "You don't promise miracle cures, and I wouldn't believe you if you did. But can you tell me what you *do* mean by 'healing'?"

"Let me try," he said. "But it's slightly different for each person, so what I tell you may sound a little broad. To me, healing is the process of experiencing greater awareness. I've also heard it defined as the integration of body and mind into the heart, or living fully in the present moment. In my experience, healing generally includes the repair of important relationships. For most people, that process includes forgiveness, acceptance, and making peace with the people who have been important to you, even if they're no longer part of your life."

"You seem to work exclusively with people who are dying," I said. "Don't you find that a little morbid?"

"I really don't," he said. "Sometimes it's sad, as you might expect, but many other emotions come into play, too, including relief and even joy. There's a great richness that often comes out when people who are facing death begin to explore the meaning of their lives. Some people with a terminal disease tend to be highly motivated, and they find that illness provides an opportunity for discovery and spiritual growth. Many of them are prepared to do difficult work, and they're not easily discouraged — even when some of the issues they're facing turn out to be complicated, demanding, or painful."

"And you've been doing this work for some time?" I asked.

"Yes. When I started out, I noticed that people with life-threatening illnesses generally fell into two camps. Many of them simply give up because their lives seem to be over, and sometimes that becomes a self-fulfilling prophecy. Other people experience their illness as a great challenge, and are so highly motivated that they're willing to consider treatments and approaches that are often dismissed as flaky or weird. Whether it's biofeedback, acupuncture, homeopathy, or the kind of mind-body work that Herb Benson does — those techniques were not widely known before the early 1970s."

When I left Rick's office and made my way back down the

stairs, I was pretty sure I had found the right therapist. And I was ready for a more holistic approach. My first experience with alternative medicine had come ten years earlier, when Dr. Benson's meditation project yielded such dramatic results. Since then I had been meditating every day. Looking back on it, I was probably a perfect candidate for some blend of the spiritual and the emotional. I was open-minded, I was rebellious, and I was already attracted to yoga and Eastern religions.

I met with Rick once a week for two years, and to some extent these sessions changed my life. He encouraged me to read books on spiritual themes that he thought I'd find helpful, such as *Love Is Letting Go of Fear* by Gerald Jampolsky; *How Shall I Live* by Richard Moss; *To Live Until We Say Good-bye* by Elisabeth Kübler-Ross; and several volumes by Stephen Levine, including *Healing into Life and Death* and *Meetings at the Edge*. I found Levine's work to be especially insightful, and I have often gone back to his books.

One of the most important techniques Rick introduced me to was guided imagery. With the help of my meditation routines and some breathing exercises, I would enter a state of deep relaxation until I found myself at a level of consciousness where my physical sensations began to fade away. I would then imagine a brilliant ball of white light floating above my head, which represented the healing energy of the universe. I would slowly allow the energy from that light to flow into the cells of my body, washing through me until I felt both its heat and its light. *Now imagine that this ball of light is transformed into a laser-like beam of white light that is directed to specific areas in your body that are in need of healing. Feel it being directed at your heart. Feel it being directed at your lungs.*

Rick prepared a tape for me, which I'd listen to at home every day. Against a background of soft, relaxing music, his soothing voice would lead me into a meditative state, where I would visualize the light and the healing beams emanating from it. Also on the tape were several affirmations that I would repeat: *I am relaxed. I am calm. I am at peace. I am whole.*

As I try to describe these sessions, I'm aware of how easily they can seem banal and simplistic, like a parody of New Age psychobabble. To some extent I share that prejudice, especially when I look back on that time from my privileged and comfortable position of good health. But I believe that when we send out positive messages about our wishes and desires, they resonate and eventually come back to us in some form — although not necessarily in the ways we may have envisioned. Almost everybody daydreams occasionally, but to do so actively and intentionally, to call up a specific vision with a sense of purpose, can provide us with encouragement, inspiration, and hope. Visualizations move us forward.

When I was suffering, these visualizations helped a lot. When you're acutely ill, and you can enter a space where you actually imagine yourself being healed, the effect can be powerful and highly therapeutic — at least to the soul. And when the soul can be healed, the body sometimes follows. But even when it doesn't, a healing soul is often its own reward.

Now I'd like you to go back in your mind's eye to a place from your childhood where you felt safe and comfortable, and to see yourself in this safe place once again. . . . I would visualize myself in a grassy field on a summer day, and the effect was so vivid and real that even during a New England winter I could feel the warm sunlight on my face.

Although my body had grown weak, I never lost my urge to dance. And here, in the secure, supportive environment of my imagination, I saw myself dancing again — whole and healthy, moving fully, passionately, and without restraint. More than once the thought occurred to me that if there really was such a thing as reincarnation, and we could somehow choose our next cycle, I would want to return as a dancer *again* — but an even better dancer this time, with more power, more passion, more grace, more agility, more of *everything*. And I would dance through my new life with even more enthusiasm than I had the first time around. I took great joy in this fantasy, never daring to believe that it would actually and literally come true in *this* lifetime.

Once, when I described these exuberant images to a friend, she asked if I didn't feel depressed or disheartened by the blatant and possibly cruel discrepancy between my waking reality and that part of my life where I was once again dancing freely. But I never did. Time after time, I found these visions uplifting and comforting. Because they took place in my own head, I was in charge; I was, in every sense, the choreographer. Had I attended a performance and seen someone *else* dancing on stage, the contrast between her physical abilities and mine would have been too painful — which is why I stopped going to dance performances, just as I had stopped going after college, when it appeared that my nascent dance career was already over. But now, in these private performances on the stage of my imagination, I was dancing as well as I had ever danced, and choreographing to music I heard in my head. I was really and fully *there,* and the healing psychological effects of these sessions remained with me long after they were over.

Although Rick was interested in a number of different treatments, not everything he suggested was helpful. Rolfing, a form of deep-tissue massage, had little effect on me. Rick had studied with Ida Rolf, who invented this technique, which involves an intense and often painful stretching of various muscles and connective tissues. The idea, which makes sense to me, is that manipulating these areas can release significant early memories that are somehow stored in the body. But for me, at least, it wasn't helpful. One of the qualities I appreciated about Rick was that he was undogmatic; he was searching, too, and he understood that not every treatment would necessarily benefit every client.

Exactly two years after it began, my stay of execution came to an end. Suddenly the stairs to Rick's office seemed steeper than usual, and the problem quickly grew worse. Although I had known all along that Procardia was only a temporary solution, I was severely disappointed when its powers began to wane. Evidently I had harbored more fantasies than I knew that this dramatic improvement in my health would continue indefinitely.

When my old symptoms began recurring, including fatigue and shortness of breath, Rick urged me to see one of his colleagues, an experienced homeopathic doctor who interviewed me at length and gave me a remedy that consisted of the venom of a poisonous South American snake. It sounded bizarre, but I was willing to try it — not only because I was feeling desperate, but also because one of my regular doctors had recently mentioned an experimental new medicine that was derived from snake venom. Okay, I thought, I'll just be taking the same prescription in its natural form. What have I got to lose?

But the treatment only exacerbated my symptoms. The following day I was supposed to go to lunch with Barbara Katz, a sculptor I had met on the local arts council. I was feeling so weak that I called Barbara to cancel, but she insisted on stopping by to check on me. It's a good thing she did, because when she entered the apartment she found me almost lifeless on the living-room couch. Barbara called an ambulance and rushed me to the hospital, where I rested for a few days until I was strong enough to go home. From my hospital room, I spoke by telephone to the homeopath, who explained that dilute solutions sometimes exaggerate the symptoms, bringing on a "healing crisis." But I was in no position to exaggerate anything, so that was it for homeopathy.

This episode seemed to hasten my decline, and during the final weeks of 1987 I was in and out of the hospital several times. On New Year's Eve, my boyfriend Alan and four of our friends came by with party hats and champagne, and this impromptu celebration really lifted my spirits. No matter how badly I was feeling, I was never too sick for a party.

But my condition was getting worse, and additional doses of Procardia had no effect. When I wasn't in the hospital, I was housebound and using oxygen. When I could no longer leave the apartment, Rick made occasional house calls.

I could feel my body sinking and shrinking, losing its muscle tone and vitality as the aging process accelerated. I started shedding years of earthly, mundane concerns — caring for the house, deciding what to cook, whom to call, and where to go, as the physical details of daily life became increasingly meaningless. I felt myself rising to another plane, a place of clarity and calm, lightness and peace. What is happening? I wondered. Is it the soul arising from the body? Is this denial? Or perhaps acceptance? Will the anger come soon?

But I was too tired for anger — or anything else. When I dropped the soap in the shower, I no longer had the strength to pick it up. Little by little, I felt myself giving up another piece of life each day. Looking at myself in the mirror, I saw old and I saw tired. I saw blue lips, fading eyes, sallow skin. Oh, Grandma, am I you?

Grandma appeared to me in a dream where she collapsed in

my arms. "It's not like I thought it would be, to die," she told me. "It's really quite wonderful." And then she expired, and while I held her, she disintegrated. A moment later she was gone, and I was left with her essence — melted wax in the palm of my hand. In the dream I thought, How wonderful. All of us, the entire world — we are all just a procession of people.

My grandmother was telling me that I didn't have to fear death. Dying is normal, it's part of life. Before his own death, my grandfather had made a similar point. "Twenty, thirty, sixty, eighty" — he was counting in Yiddish — "vat the hell's the difference? You live and you die."

I had never thought much about my own death, and even now I was far more focused on staying alive. But death had become part of my reality, and from time to time I did think about it. My fear about dying was connected to not understanding it, and not really being able to imagine that I would no longer exist. Was it like sleep, I wondered, where my body is still there but I'm not conscious? Would the world really keep going after I was gone? I knew the answer, of course, but it was still a difficult concept to grasp. How can we possibly understand our own nonexistence?

It was easier to focus on my funeral. I wanted to be cremated, with my ashes scattered in the ocean. Instead of mourning my death, I wanted the guests to celebrate my life with champagne, gardenias, and Beethoven. After all, most funerals have a celebratory component, and after the service, friends and relatives often share food and companionship. An actual celebration might be a little jarring, but I did like the idea of throwing one last party — even if I could be there only in spirit.

As I grew weaker, my sense of time started to change. On the one hand, I probably didn't have all that much of it left. On the other hand, time was just about all I *did* have. Sitting still or lying in bed, I was acutely aware of the ticking of the clock, and of the many tasks and activities, both interesting and ordinary, that were no longer filling the hours of each day. I felt an odd blending of floating in endless time while also being aware that my earthly time was limited. I was living in a kind of dimensionless present.

For the first time in my life, I had no real future to look forward to. I had always assumed that when the time finally came to face death I'd be a much older woman, in my seventies or eighties. But now, what I had previously envisioned as my middle years had abruptly been transformed into my curtain call. You're supposed to be *old* at the end of your life, but I was only forty-seven!

While my contemporaries were going through their midlife crises, I was fading away. Or maybe I was having the ultimate midlife crisis, where midlife and end-life were unfolding simultaneously. And yet I don't remember feeling angry that I was being cheated out of two or three entire decades that most people my age could look forward to. This was the hand I was dealt, and I would play it as best I could.

Sometimes the days and nights merged into one. Lying in bed, I would occasionally wonder: if I close my eyes and fall asleep, how can I be sure I'll wake up? Each breath I took might be my last, and sometimes the sound of my own gasps wrenched me out of my light sleep. How long, I wondered, can I go on like this?

I was continually aware of Amara in the next room. Was she sleeping, or was she lying awake and crying again? By now, of course, she knew everything; how could there possibly be any secrets between us? She was crying a lot, and she couldn't hide her sadness or her fear.

I had some idea of how difficult it was for Amara to come into my room and see me like this: floating in my bed, my color gone, and an oxygen tube in my nose. But I was so focused on my own situation, and so accustomed to it, that I didn't always realize how painful it must have been. My illness was the overriding reality of *her* life, too, and she had started writing about my condition in some of her school assignments. One paper, from early 1988, began: "Claire Sylvia lies on her bed, looking relaxed and quite comfortable even though she has an oxygen tank next to her. . . ." And it continued: "Because of her illness she's unable to do most anything that will take her energy away. This brings pain to her face."

Poor girl, having to write these words. Who was attending to the pain in *her* face? In her papers she expressed more emotion than she ever let me see.

Amara was almost sixteen now, and increasingly independent. I no longer had the strength to impose curfews or other forms of discipline. Like many single parents, I tended to be overly lenient in any case, and the vivid, painful memories of my own tyrannical mother made me even more indulgent. But now there was so much I didn't know, so much I couldn't do. I no longer knew who her friends were, and I couldn't even attend Open School night, when the parents were invited to meet their children's teachers. Because Amara was already burdened by my illness, I hired a part-time housekeeper to help out with shopping, cooking, cleaning, and laundry.

I knew that Amara had a boyfriend, but I discovered only later that for a long time she hadn't let him know how sick I really was. For months, Danny's parents had wondered why I never drove Amara anywhere. When they finally learned the truth, they welcomed Amara into their family and were incredibly supportive to me.

I also didn't realize that my illness was putting an enormous strain on Amara's relationship with Danny. She couldn't complain to me, so she opened up to him. But like many high school boys, Danny wasn't yet mature enough to provide the emotional support that Amara needed. They often fought, although Amara understood that she wasn't so much angry at Danny as upset about her mother. Their relationship began to deteriorate, and soon Amara found herself making deals with God: "Okay, I'll give up my boyfriend if you save my mother's life." I'm glad I didn't know about this until much later.

I twice tried to take Amara on a cruise, but both times we had to cancel because I was too sick to travel. And when the Procardia was still working, I had bought advance tickets to *Les Misérables*. I was looking forward to taking Amara for her sixteenth birthday, but when February came around I was too sick to go. I felt terrible: for most of Amara's life there had been only two of us in our little family, and now, increasingly, there was only one. I recalled my own unhappy adolescence, when our family of four felt small and unhappy. This was even worse.

Sometimes I'd wake up in the morning and tell myself that I simply must have a shower today. Then I'd realize that I probably ought to wait until someone else was in the house, because taking a shower wasn't something I should be doing alone — just in case. But there were so *many* "just in case's."

In case what? I pass out? I go numb again? That had already happened: I was in the car when my whole left side suddenly went numb and I had to pull off the road. That was it for driving.

What was the worst that could happen? I could die, of course, which was probably just a matter of time. Dying was no longer confined to the future; it could happen any day, any hour.

When would it be? What would it feel like? Who would discover me? Would it be Amara? And what would that do to my poor baby?

The questions never stopped. Time to calm myself. Time to meditate, to move from the physical to the spiritual.

Spirituality is one of those amorphous terms that means different things to different people. I like Bernie Siegel's definition: the ability to find peace and happiness in an imperfect world. Fortunately, I was able to find some of each. Despite everything I was facing, I never had suicidal thoughts. I understand the impulse, but I'm opposed to the act. I believe that each of us is given a life, and however long or painful that life may be, ending it is God's decision, not ours. We can't presume to know what God has in mind for us. But in all fairness, I can imagine feeling differently if I suffered from intolerable pain. Fortunately, I never did.

No matter how bad things were, I was usually able to move my thoughts in a more positive direction. Maybe there's no such thing as dying, I told myself at one point. Maybe you're either living or you're dead. And if that's the case, I'm definitely alive. For a while that idea was comforting — that even if I was 90 percent dead, that meant I was still 10 percent alive, which put me on the right side of the equation.

Throughout these months I remembered Mary Gohlke's words of encouragement: Keep going, I told myself, breath by breath, moment by moment, no matter how hard it gets. Keep breathing, even if you have to pretend to breathe. Finding myself in this grave situation, I dared not think macabre thoughts, of corpses, funerals, eulogies, and coffins.

Keep going! Don't give up, I told myself. You're still part of the world. Life is still flowing everywhere around you. And even, however faintly, within you.

Five

Difficult Days

VALENTINE'S DAY, 1988. Just when it seemed that things couldn't get worse, Alan left me. We had been together for seven good years, and ever since Mary Gohlke's *Parade* article, when my life changed forever, he had cared for me and helped me with hundreds of worldly details I could no longer attend to. But now, after pulling away for several weeks, he was gone. First the Procardia ran out of steam, and then Alan.

I was devastated. With Alan gone, I felt a terrible loneliness. I had made my peace with dying, but now I was abandoned. In all probability, I would be ending my life alone. Although I had known that Alan might leave, I was miserable when it actually happened.

The nights were the hardest. For five years Alan and I had spent virtually every night together, which was longer than some marriages — including one of mine. This was the hardest time of my life. The misery of being dumped is bad enough, but under normal circumstances you can at least imagine or hope that some day love will find you again. In my condition, that seemed extremely unlikely.

Thank God for my friend Barbara Katz, who was fast becoming my guardian angel. In January, when the transplant people at

Johns Hopkins had agreed to see me for an evaluation, I was too weak to travel to Baltimore by myself. Alan hadn't offered to take me, and by then I couldn't bring myself to ask. Although our friendship was still new, Barbara stepped right in.

In Baltimore, I was given a series of tests to monitor my heart and lungs. The doctors even examined my fingertips and my nails to determine how much oxygen was getting through to my extremities. But while the medical staff was very considerate, they were careful not to paint too rosy a picture about the operation I was there to discuss. "A transplant is a mixed blessing," said one of the nurses. "To some extent, you'll just be exchanging one set of problems for another."

That's easy for you to say, I thought. At least I'd be alive to *have* a set of problems.

I had gone to Hopkins with a mixture of hope and skepticism, and while we were there I felt pulled in both directions. I was hoping they would list me as a candidate, and to my great relief, they did. But they also made clear that it might well take a year or even two years before I was called, which was something I had already learned from my research and networking.

But even if I lived long enough for the call to come in, I wasn't sure how I would respond. While a transplant would probably save my life, it was still an enormously frightening and dangerous operation. Was this really something that I could do? I honestly didn't know. I was applying for membership in a society I didn't necessarily want to join.

While I expected that my evaluation would include various tests and measurements, I hadn't realized that the transplant team was just as interested in my character and my outlook. Understandably, they saw themselves as guardians of a precious gift that was in exceedingly short supply, and to be blunt about it, they weren't about to waste that gift on anyone who wasn't a good bet to take excellent care of it. When you perform enough transplants, they told me, the operation itself becomes almost routine. More often than not, what ultimately determines a patient's survival is what happens in the months and years after the surgery.

While some of the variables are beyond anyone's control, one key factor that affects survival rates is the recipient's subsequent behavior and her willingness to accept responsibility. "We can transplant almost anyone," I was told. "But because there are many more applicants than donors, we look for people with a high potential for compliance. We can't monitor the patients after they leave the hospital, so we're looking for people who will be scrupulous about taking their medications, following the necessary precautions, and returning at regular intervals for follow-up visits."

They were also interested in candidates who had a positive, life-affirming attitude. While I evidently scored high on that scale, it was clear that a few eyebrows had been raised by my recent experiment with snake venom — which, I was sorry to learn, had already become part of my medical records. Even so, my motivation and my will to live came through loud and clear.

I returned home from Hopkins with more hope than I had felt in months. I also brought back a pair of beepers that were supposed to alert me — or my partner, in case I missed the signal — in the event that a suitable heart and lungs suddenly became available. At that point, assuming I said yes, Amara and I would drop everything and fly down to Baltimore on a private jet.

I was too weak to leave the house, but Amara wore her beeper everywhere, including school. Nobody had warned us that these devices sometimes go off accidentally, and while my beeper was silent, Amara had to cope with three or four false alarms over the next few months, all of them during class. Each time the beeper went off, she'd go tearing down the halls to call me. I would immediately call Hopkins, where the transplant team would say "No, sorry, it must be a mistake." Then I'd call Amara at the school office to tell her there was no news. This process must have been awful for her, and I can only imagine how vulnerable she felt each time it happened.

It was easier for me. Some people on transplant waiting lists become obsessed with their beepers, but I didn't give it much thought. Whether I was ever called for a transplant was totally out of my hands, and somehow I was able to accept that. I now believe that not having decided whether to accept the offer — assuming, of course, that it ever came — made waiting a little easier. Postponing this decision was my way of maintaining a measure of control.

To the extent it was possible, I spent my days living as fully as I could, rather than waiting for news. Sometimes I became frightened or anxious, but when that happened, I usually had ways of coping. Between meditation, visualization, a few close friends, and an occasional Valium, I was generally able to keep my spirits up.

But not always. There were times when I wanted to scream, when I wished I had the physical ability to really howl. Sometimes, when I was using oxygen, I was seized by a powerful desire to rip the cord off my nose and to run out the door and into a field. This was followed by a stifling claustrophobia when it hit me again that I couldn't do that. There were times when I thought I'd go out of my mind with frustration and fear.

When friends and acquaintances heard I was on the waiting list for a transplant at Hopkins, they started congratulating me as if I had won an award or passed an important audition. I could never get used to this, and I still find it weird. Imagine: a hospital has agreed, at least in principle, to rip the heart and lungs out of your body and replace them with the heart and lungs of somebody who has just died. And for this you're being congratulated?

Today, of course, being wait-listed for a transplant is a little more common. It wouldn't surprise me if Hallmark has issued a greeting card that begins "So you're having a transplant!"

While Alan's departure was a terrible blow, I also felt some relief when he left. Now I no longer had to worry about being too much of a burden. Several other friends fell away, too. For some people, being around a dying person is too painful a reminder of their own mortality, or is otherwise so difficult that it's often better for both sides if they simply withdraw — at least for a while. That way, the negative energy leaves with them.

While some friends vanished, others appeared to fill the vacuum. My nephew Stuart, Marilyn's son, was a frequent visitor and a terrific companion. Barbara looked in on me often, while two other friends, Ruth and Anita, brought me dinners, ran errands, and came by almost every day. Even when there were no errands to be done, it felt good to know that some people wanted to be with me.

At first, however, these visits were difficult in a way I hadn't anticipated. I felt awkward and guilty at being so incapacitated, and so dependent on my friends. Before I could fully appreciate their generosity, I had to learn how to accept help. I had always been more comfortable as the caretaker, and at first it felt disconcerting to find myself on the receiving end of these loving transactions.

I also had to accept the simple reality that there were many simple tasks I could no longer do for myself, including silly little things that were either unnecessary or compulsive, such as putting every last item in its proper place, or organizing the magazines on the coffee table in just the right way. With a little practice and a lot of willpower, I was gradually able to surrender some of my desire for neatness, order, and control. But I never got used to having other people, even close friends, puttering around in my kitchen.

Sometimes I wondered: How can I possibly repay the friends who came to me with such love and compassion? Eventually, I understood that I *was* giving something back, simply by welcoming and appreciating their efforts. Giving and generosity, I realized, are as therapeutic and helpful to the giver as they are to the recipient. When I put myself in their position, I realized that they genuinely wanted to help, or even needed to. And when I understood that in some subtle way I *was* giving something back to those who gave to me, I stopped feeling sorry for myself. To be a graceful and appreciative recipient is in itself a kind of gift to the giver.

Without saying so explicitly, my visitors made it clear that this was indeed a two-way transaction, and that in giving to me, they were also learning from me. Later on, when I cared for other people who were very sick, I learned this lesson for myself: that when you spend time with people who are dying, you discover a lot about living. These visits can be stressful and arduous, but they can also be enormously rewarding. Even as my physical self was shrinking, my spiritual self was expanding.

But I still wanted to acknowledge my friends in a more tangible way, and one morning the idea occurred to me to throw a small party for the people who were so good to me. Coming to my apartment had become a pretty grim experience, and at least once, I wanted my visitors to have a happy time in my presence, and with each other. While it felt a little strange to be planning a celebration, I found that just thinking about the details — the food, the music, the guest list — gave me an energizing dose of pleasure and strength. To some small extent, I was being *me* again — entertaining, organizing, bringing people together. At a time when so many pieces of my identity were disappearing, it was wonderful to be planning a party.

I had help of course, especially from Amara, who prepared the food. I also ordered a big cake inscribed with the phrase "To Life." Some of my friends brought *their* friends and partners, and Amara invited a couple of her own friends as well. I stayed with the group as long as I was able, and then retired to my room with my oxygen tank to enjoy the happy sounds of laughter. The party was just what I had hoped for. When I die, I thought, this is how I'd like my funeral to be.

Barbara told me years later that she thought this party marked a turning point. "You had every reason to give up," she told me, "but here you were making a statement, just like the phrase on that cake, that you intended not only to survive, but to *live*." Barbara was probably right. I had assumed this party was for my friends, but of course it was also for me.

Sometimes, when there were no errands to be done and nothing that required conversation, my visitors would just sit quietly with me. Their presence was always comforting, and often healing. They knew they couldn't take my pain away, and they made no effort to distract me, or themselves, with talk, gifts, or other diversions. When I was too weak to speak, or was otherwise inclined toward quiet, I was always grateful for visitors who understood that silence, too, is a form of communication. When I danced with Helen Tamiris, she would occasionally remind us that keeping perfectly still during a dance routine is itself a form of movement, just as a brief silence or rest during a piece of music is a vital part of the total musical expression.

These days, whenever I go to see a friend in the hospital, I notice that many visitors are busy filling the air with a constant stream of chatter, or are restlessly flitting around the room. With the best of intentions, people tend to regard silence or stillness as an embarrassment, or an enemy to be obliterated at every opportunity. So my advice to those who are visiting sick friends or relatives: you don't always need to speak. The mere fact that you are *there*, in the room, may convey everything that needs to be communicated.

But there were also times when the words of my visitors were extremely helpful. I was in the hospital one evening when my friends Judy and Derek came to visit. They arrived at a moment when I was particularly weak and frightened. My blood pressure had dropped dramatically, and the alarmed nurse had gone to look for the doctor. Judy told me later that one of the nurses had said, "Claire's lungs are like tissue paper, and we're having trouble finding a pulse."

As I gazed at the door, Judy appeared. She came quickly to the bed, enfolded me in her arms, and began to pray for me and with me. I totally let go to her, to the prayers, and to God as I had never done before. She must have held me tightly for half an hour, and tears were washing my face. She was like a mother holding a child, a holding I had needed and wanted all my life. I couldn't remember ever being held that way by my own mother.

Judy and Derek are Christian Scientists, and Judy was reciting — well, not just reciting, but really *praying* — the words of a well-known poem by Mary Baker Eddy called "Mother's Evening Prayer." It begins:

> *O gentle presence, peace and joy and power;*
> *O Life divine, that owns each waiting hour,*

Thou Love that guards the nestling's faltering flight!
Keep Thou my child on upward wing tonight.

Love is our refuge; only with mine eye
Can I behold the snare, the pit, the fall:
His habitation high is here, and nigh,
His arm encircles me, and mine, and all.

As Judy prayed with me that evening, I felt myself being held in God's right hand. Judy grew up knowing God as both Father and Mother, and during her prayer I experienced both of these powerful images.

As Judy was praying, her husband Derek came into the room. When Judy was finished, Derek took my hand and recited the Twenty-third Psalm, "The Lord Is My Shepherd." I had heard these words all my life, but now, in this context, they were almost burning with meaning.

Yea, though I walk through the valley of the shadow of death, I will fear no evil, for Thou art with me.

That night, I knew, He really was with me.

Rainbow Connection

IN APRIL, some promising news: Yale–New Haven Hospital in Connecticut was about to become the fourth medical center in the country, and the first in New England, to perform heart-lung transplants. The new program was being built around Dr. John Baldwin, a rising star in the world of transplant surgery, who had previously been at Stanford. Yale was an easy drive from Boston, and it was encouraging to know that another potential lifeline might soon be available. My doctor shared my optimism; he promised to write to Dr. Baldwin to ask if I could be evaluated at Yale.

In early May, I awoke one morning feeling particularly frail. When I called my doctor to see whether he had heard from Dr. Baldwin, his secretary informed me that he had just left the country for three weeks. When I specifically asked about the new transplant program at Yale, she said my doctor hadn't yet contacted them on my behalf.

It took all my energy just to make that call. If I'd had any strength to spare, I would have been furious that nothing had happened. Instead, I closed my eyes and drifted off to sleep.

Once again Barbara rescued me; this was getting to be a

habit. When she came to see me that afternoon, I was weaker than ever. "You looked *green,*" she said later.

I told her my doctor hadn't even written to Yale.

"I'm not surprised," she said. Barbara had met him two or three times when I was in the hospital, and she was convinced he had given up on me. Now she began to take on the anger that I was too exhausted to feel.

"I'm calling Yale," she said, reaching for the phone.

"But they don't have my records."

"I'm calling anyway. We can't just sit here and let you fade away."

Whether it was luck, persistence, or providence, Barbara got right through to the person in charge. Gail Eddy was the coordinator of Yale's new transplant program, and after Barbara described my situation, Gail asked to speak to me.

"I think you should come for an evaluation," she said. "Don't worry about your records; I'll have them sent. When can you be here?"

It was an odd question, because I had nothing on my calendar for the rest of my life. Could I come down in two weeks? Definitely. Now all I had to do was stay alive until then, which suddenly didn't seem all that difficult. Maybe I was kidding myself, but my brief conversation with Gail Eddy had given me hope.

My unconscious mind must have felt the same way, for that night I had two auspicious dreams. In the first one, a sharp, shiny knife floated in front of me, surrounded by a white glow. As I watched in amazement, the knife cut the neck of a baby, near his Adam's apple. But I knew the baby wasn't hurt, because there was no crying and no blood.

In the second dream, the transplant was already over. It had gone smoothly, with no pain, and right after the operation I was walking around. But the doctors hadn't told me that I would need to drink four glasses of milk each day. I learned this by chance, talking to somebody else.

It seemed clear that both dreams were strongly optimistic projections about the transplant. In the first one, the operation was painless and almost otherworldly. I was the baby — a male baby, for some reason. In the second dream I was myself, although the four glasses of milk did suggest a baby or a small child. In both dreams, the operation had been successful.

A week later, I had a third and more elaborate dream. I was pregnant, but my skin was translucent, which allowed me to see the baby within. It looked like a little E.T. figure as it waved its tiny hand. But the baby's face was the face of my mother. I was about to give birth to my own mother!

In this dream, I realized later, the extraterrestrial creature was greeting me from his capsule in my inner world. Although he hadn't yet arrived, he was holding up the open hand of friendship. He was my child, a harbinger of my new, post-transplant self. But he was also my mother. In effect, I was carrying the embryo that would give birth to my new life.

But why E.T.? Perhaps because E.T. was a creature of the heart. Late in the movie he appears to die, but when his "people" arrive to rescue him, his heart lights up and he returns to life. Perhaps this image of rebirth and resurrection was a dream echo of *Giselle* and *Limelight*.

Later on, I would examine these dreams more closely. But for now, my short-term goal was to make it to the evaluation. Until then, I went to sleep each night with my standard two-part prayer: that I would wake up the next morning, and that I would somehow survive beyond that — long enough to be there for Amara, at least until she finished high school.

*　　*　　*

The evaluation at Yale was shorter and simpler than the one at Hopkins, which was just as well, because I could barely make it from the wheelchair to the examining table. I spent most of the day with Gail Eddy, a bright, upbeat, and vivacious woman with long blond hair, blue eyes, and a terrific smile. I liked her enormously, and we seemed to have an immediate rapport.

Gail, who had previously worked as an intensive care nurse at this same hospital, brought me in to meet Dr. Baldwin, and the two of them interviewed me in a small office. It was strange, given the circumstances, but I felt as if I were interviewing them, too. Although I had heard that Dr. Baldwin was in his late thirties, I was struck by his boyish face. At the same time, he projected an aura of considerable self-confidence. He told me that at Stanford he had performed forty-nine heart-lung transplants. If he was trying to reassure me, it worked.

Like their counterparts at Hopkins, Gail and Dr. Baldwin asked about my family, my medical history, and my reasons for seeking a transplant. At the end of the interview, Dr. Baldwin said, "In my view, you're sick enough to be listed, along with three other candidates whom we have already seen. At the moment, the program hasn't officially opened; we're still waiting for permission from the state. But we expect it soon, and the moment it comes through, we'll list you." Here, too, I was reminded that it often takes a year or two before a suitable donor is found, and that an appropriate match depends, among other factors, on compatible blood types and organ size. Even so, I left Yale feeling that my chances of staying alive had just doubled. Gail had a similar reaction. "I'm going to be seeing that woman again," she told her secretary.

Back in my apartment the next morning, I read through the patient handbook that Gail had given me, which spelled out some of the nitty-gritty details of heart-lung transplants. Barbara came over in the afternoon, and because she had been with me at Hopkins, she was especially eager to hear about my trip to Yale. We were in my kitchen, eating chocolate cake with vanilla ice cream, when the phone rang. Amara usually answered, but she was in the shower, so I picked it up.

"Claire? It's Gail Eddy. Seventeen hours ago, just after you left, we received permission to open the program. We listed you right away, and we have a donor for you today."

The phone was silent as she awaited my reaction. But I was speechless. I couldn't think of anything to say.

This can't be happening, I thought. I was there only yesterday, hoping to get on a list that didn't even exist yet. This was weird. It seemed to have a "meant-to-be" quality.

"We figure you've got about two hours to get back here. How about it, Claire?"

Omigod, Omigod. This is unbelievable! My mind started racing through half a zillion thoughts, none of which I could articulate. All the things I would need to arrange. What I would bring. Here I was, facing a sudden, life-and-death decision, and what was I thinking about? My hair! Thank God I just had it cut. But did I shave my legs?

"What do you say, Claire?"

I still couldn't answer. I was overwhelmed as I tried to comprehend the magnitude and meaning of this amazing gift.

Barbara was right beside me. I looked at her and said, "What should I do?"

But my decision had already been made. I just needed support.

"Go for it," Barbara said.

Still unable to answer Gail, I handed the phone to Barbara.

Just then Amara came running out of the shower, dripping wet. Somehow she knew what was happening. "Tell her yes!" I called to Barbara as Amara and I hugged through our tears. For months, we'd each had a suitcase packed and ready to go, in case Hopkins came through.

Barbara handed me the phone, and the next few minutes were right out of an old screwball comedy. Barbara is nearly blind, and I was on oxygen, connected by a long cord to a tank in the bedroom. The two of us were passing the phone back and forth, asking questions, yelling instructions, and tripping over furniture. Twice we disconnected the call entirely, and Gail, completely calm, had to call back. Amara was busily making calls on her own line, while Gail was also arranging for a helicopter to take me to Yale.

"What should I bring?" I asked her.

"Sneakers, shorts, and a tee-shirt."

"No, seriously!"

"I *am* serious. You're going to be up on an exercise bike right after the operation."

Yeah, right. But I packed them anyway. By now I was hyperventilating from all the excitement, and I swallowed half a Valium to calm myself down.

Gail told me to meet the helicopter at a landing pad near the Museum of Fine Arts. But it was a humid day and I was having trouble breathing. The helicopter had no air conditioning, and it was so small that neither Amara nor Barbara would be able to come with me. I asked Gail if there were any other options.

"I guess you could drive," she said. "But you'll have to leave right away, and you should alert the state police that you'll be going pretty fast."

By now the Valium was kicking in, and I became calmer. I knew how I wanted this trip to proceed: I would travel by car with Amara and Barbara. I was willing to sacrifice speed if it meant a little comfort and support.

Barbara called her husband to see if he could drive us. Remarkably, she caught Bob just as he was leaving the house; another few seconds and he would have been gone. Bob said he'd be right over — another good sign.

Moments later, we were on the road: Bob and Barbara were in the front seat; Amara, my oxygen tank, and I were in the back. As the car glided toward New Haven, I lay down with my feet on Amara's lap. I had brought along a meditation tape to calm me down, and it helped. Despite all the excitement, I was feeling at peace. Between meditation and Valium, I was covering all my bets.

We had been driving for about an hour when Amara tapped me on the leg and pointed to the side window. "Look, Mom!" There, peeking out of the clouds, was the brightest, most beautiful rainbow I had ever seen. I smiled at Amara, and our eyes met, both of us silently sharing the knowledge that this was a good omen. I took my daughter's hand and squeezed it. This was our rainbow connection.

Bob's turbo-charged Chrysler LeBaron had a big digital speedometer, and at one point, Amara told me later, she noticed with alarm that we were zooming down Route 91 at 91 miles per hour. How appropriate, she thought, but how awful if Mom dies in an accident on the way to her transplant.

It was seven o'clock as we pulled up to the hospital entrance. Gail was waiting for us with a nurse and a wheelchair.

"You again?" she said with a grin.

"You know how it is," I replied. "I just couldn't stay away."

She smiled at me. "Well, as long as you're here, we might as well go upstairs. I believe they're expecting you."

*   *   *

Wasting no time, Gail helped me into the wheelchair and brought me straight to the surgical unit. A team of nurses hooked me up to an IV and gave me my first dose of cyclosporine, an antirejection drug.* From my reading, I knew that if all went well I would be taking this medicine for the rest of my life. Cyclosporine is so important in organ transplants that the first order of business was to make sure I wasn't allergic to it.

Although we had rushed like crazy to get to the hospital, it soon became clear that the actual transplant was still a few hours away. The medical team that travels to retrieve the donated organs doesn't leave the recipient's hospital until the doctors have determined that the recipient is free of infection and

---

* Rejection is the single biggest problem in organ transplants. Somehow our cells are able to detect the presence of any element that, in the body's opinion, doesn't belong there. When an unidentified intruder shows up on its radar screen, the body's instinctive response is to treat it as an enemy agent that must be repelled, isolated, or destroyed. If the perceived intruder is a transplanted organ, the ensuing assault can lead to organ failure — and death.

Trying to prevent rejection is enormously difficult, because under normal circumstances rejection is what enables our bodies to fight off and resist a wide variety of toxins and infections that might otherwise harm us. When our immune system isn't functioning properly, or when it's suppressed by antirejection drugs, even a minor infection can have deadly consequences.

In the future, the threat of post-transplant rejection will likely be solved by imprinting the recipient's genes into the transplanted organ. The body will then perceive the new organ as familiar rather than hostile, and will therefore leave it alone.

For the moment, however, the problem of rejection is being resolved through cyclosporine. More than any other medicine, cyclosporine reduces the chances that the recipient's body will reject a transplanted organ, but without predisposing the patient to too great a likelihood of infection.

strong enough to survive the operation. Because I had been evaluated only yesterday, I didn't require a long examination. But the nurses were drawing what seemed like my entire blood supply, which would be tested and analyzed before the transplant could be done.

Like so much of life, this seemed to be a case of "hurry up and wait." But I was well aware of how fortunate I was to be here at all. I wasn't alone, either. In addition to Barbara, Bob, and Amara, who would all be spending the night at a nearby hotel, my sister Marilyn had driven up from New York with two of her sons. And although I had met her only yesterday, Gail's presence was enormously reassuring.

The scene that night was slightly surreal and more than a little ironic: although I was awaiting a dramatic and dangerous operation, I felt like the guest of honor at a party. My hospital room was filled with love. At one point, looking up at all the concerned faces around me, I actually felt sad for my visitors in the event that I didn't survive.

I certainly hadn't expected to be feeling at ease at this moment, but if serenity was within reach, I was happy to embrace it. I knew perfectly well where I was and what I was facing, but I wasn't worried. If this turned out to be my final night on earth, so be it. I felt no press of unfinished business, no agenda of words left unsaid.

All the meditations, visualizations, and important conversations I had been part of in the past couple of years seemed to culminate in this moment. It reminded me of that moment in dance when I would gather up my combined resources of mind, body, and spirit, and risk all as I stepped onto the ball of one foot and plunged into a long arabesque. As a dancer, I knew what it felt like to extend every part of my being into unknown space. You arrive at a moment in time and space when you believe you will succeed, and that all your work has prepared you to risk everything. And you fly.

Once or twice that evening, my mind flashed back to the dreams I'd had three weeks ago, in which I had already survived the transplant. Those dreams felt real to me now, and I hoped they were prophetic. One of them, it seemed, already was: earlier, when the nurse had given me my first dose of cyclosporine, she had put the medicine in a cup of chocolate milk and had explained that I would be taking two such doses a day, each with two cups of milk. In the dream, I had been told that I would be drinking four cups of milk a day.

The one thing that made me anxious was that this would be the first heart-lung transplant ever done in New England. Other than Dr. Baldwin, everybody on the medical team would be going through this procedure for the first time. I felt like a pioneer, which was both exciting and scary. But I also remembered that Dr. Baldwin had performed this operation dozens of times at Stanford, and that I was in excellent hands.

I was feeling spacey from the Valium, and from at least one of the drugs that was coming through the IV. I tried to put all of my thoughts together into one positive visualization of a successful outcome, but right now I couldn't manage it. The medication was plunging me into a swirling, half-awake dream state that fragmented my thoughts and made concentration impossible.

One of the medications was drying out my mouth. Because I couldn't eat or drink before the operation, my only option was to suck on a damp washcloth. But I was feeling so woozy that I had trouble getting it to my mouth. Amara sat with me, and both of us were laughing as she helped me negotiate the washcloth's long and treacherous journey from my hand to my face.

I was grateful for the literature Gail had given me yesterday at the evaluation. Was it really only *yesterday*? Just this morning

I had read that after the operation, when the anesthesia wore off and I woke up, an endotracheal breathing tube in my windpipe would prevent me from speaking, and my hands would be tied to prevent me from pulling out the tube. The breathing tube would be connected to a respirator, which would be breathing for me during and immediately after the surgery. Somehow, knowing this in advance felt important to me.

Finally it was time for my visitors to leave. When Marilyn leaned over to kiss me goodbye, I could see the tears in her eyes. "I just thought of something," she said. "If you can't talk after the operation, how will we know you're all right?"

I told her that when I woke up, if everything was okay I would wink at her.

In my final lucid moments, through the fog of the tranquilizer and the other medications, Gail came in with Dr. Hammond, the assisting surgeon, to let me know they would soon be leaving to "harvest" the organs. That word startled me. I had never heard it used this way, and it has since been replaced by other, more agreeable terms, such as "retrieve" or "procure." I noticed that Dr. Hammond was wearing high boots and suspenders, which made him look like a man about to leave on a fishing trip. In a way, I suppose he was.

Gail explained that while she and Dr. Hammond were gone, Dr. Baldwin would remain with me in the hospital. He would begin the operation as soon as he was notified that the donor's heart and lungs had been removed, but Gail assured me that he wouldn't remove my own heart and lungs until the new organs — *my* new organs — had made it safely back to the operating room in New Haven.

But by this time I was far too groggy to focus on these grotesque and horrifying details, which was probably just as well. Nor did I fully understand that at one point in the process my body would be without *any* heart and lungs, and that during this time I would be kept alive by a machine. That was too bizarre to contemplate.

Dr. Baldwin came in and said, "We're going to put you under now. Claire, I have to remind you that it's always possible that something could go wrong, and the organs won't arrive in good condition. This sometimes happens with the lungs, which are very fragile. They could be damaged or bruised during transit. We expect to do this transplant, but sometimes, at the very last minute, things just don't work out."

I looked up at him and said, "That's okay. Do what you have to. It's in God's hands now."

I meant it. That night, too, I felt the presence of God. And I truly believed that God would be working through the hands of the surgeons and nurses who were with the donor in Maine, and who would be with me in this hospital in Connecticut.

It was three in the morning when they finally brought me to the operating room. Dr. Baldwin's words of caution were the last thing I heard before falling into a deep sleep.

Seven

While
I Was Out

IT HAD BEGUN with a phone call. While Barbara and I were sitting in my kitchen, the Maine coordinator from the New England Organ Bank called Gail at her office. The organ bank was already aware of my blood type, tissue type, and body size. "We have a donor for Claire Sylvia," the coordinator told Gail. "A male, eighteen. He's brain-dead,* and the family has given consent. Cause of death was a head injury from a motorcycle accident. We are now placing organs, and the heart and lungs are suitable for donation. We have a normal echocardiogram, good left ventricular function, normal valve, normal heart. The patient had no CPR." The coordinator listed various other facts and figures, which Gail dutifully recorded.

"I'll call you right back," she said.

When the call had come in, Dr. Baldwin was in surgery, doing a heart bypass. Gail suited up and entered the operating room, where she informed him that a donor was available for Claire Sylvia — a young man with a good medical history, no

---

* A brain-dead patient is one in whom all brain activity has ceased forever, but whose heart is still beating — either naturally or artificially. Legally, the patient is dead.

heart disease, and normal heart and lungs. She read him all the values and measurements from the coordinator.

"Accept the organs," Dr. Baldwin said. The numbers were good and Gail could see that he was pleased. She called the man from the organ bank and said yes. Then she called me.

While I was on my way to New Haven, Gail arranged for a Learjet to fly a medical team from Yale–New Haven Hospital to a medical center in Maine, where they would remove the donor's heart and lungs and, assuming the organs were in good condition, bring them back to Connecticut. The donor's lungs had already been measured, but just to be safe, the team from Yale would be bringing along an X-ray of my lungs, which would be superimposed over an X-ray of the donor's lungs to make sure the sizes were indeed compatible.

Takeoff was scheduled for 11 P.M. In addition to Gail and Dr. Hammond, the team included four other members: a second heart surgeon; an anesthesiologist to "manage" the donor with the appropriate medications; a pump profusionist to help run chemical solutions through the donor's lungs; and a scrub nurse to assist the surgeons.

At 10:30, half an hour before takeoff, the team gathered in the operating room, where they assembled all the equipment, medications, and organ preservation solutions they might conceivably need in Maine. Because organ retrieval is often done in smaller hospitals, surgeons from the recipient's hospital generally bring their own instruments and supplies. Gail's equipment included the plastic Igloo picnic cooler that, if all went well, would hold the organs during the flight back. She had bought it at Caldor's, after discreetly holding up a tape measure to a number of different coolers until she found one that was the right size for a human heart and lungs — with a little extra room for a container and for ice.

At 10:45 P.M., an ambulance met the team at the entrance to the emergency room and drove them to a waiting jet at Tweed Airport in East Haven. Throughout the afternoon and evening, Gail had been in telephone contact with the coordinator in Maine to ensure that the donor's condition remained stable. So far his lungs were still oxygenating well, and his chest X-ray looked clear. Earlier on, before any of the organs were made available, the donor's blood had been tested to determine its type, and to ensure there was no sign of the HIV virus, hepatitis, or any other infection. The donor was being maintained on a ventilator, which breathed for him; his heart, however, was still beating on its own. But because a brain-dead patient can quickly become unstable, there was no time to lose.

As the team from Yale made its way to Maine, two other teams were flying to Maine from hospitals in Boston to retrieve the donor's kidneys and his liver. Of all organ transplant teams, the heart-lung group must cope with the shortest amount of *ischemic* time, which measures how long the organs can survive with no blood or oxygen. From removal in Maine to implantation in Connecticut, the team had no more than four hours.

As soon as the team landed in Maine, an ambulance met them on the runway and rushed them to the donor's hospital. The two pilots would remain at the airport, and Gail had their phone number in the event of an unexpected change in schedule. Retrieval teams are sometimes delayed when a small hospital's sole operating room must suddenly be used for emergency surgery. Tonight, however, everything went smoothly. As the procedure was nearing an end, Gail would call the pilots with an estimated departure time so they could be waiting on the runway with the door open.

As soon as the ambulance reached the hospital, the team from Yale went straight to the Intensive Care Unit, where the two surgeons studied the donor's chart and reviewed his history. So far, everything looked fine. Gail called New Haven to report that the donor was about to be moved to the operating room.

In the OR, the anesthesiologist made sure the donor was given the correct intravenous fluids and medications. The surgeons then opened the donor's chest with a sternal saw and inspected the heart and lungs. This was a critical moment, because certain injuries and diseases don't always show up on X-rays or tests. The surgeons had flown to Maine not only to retrieve the organs, but to determine for themselves that the heart and lungs were healthy and in good condition.

After the inspection, the surgeons backed away from the table and made room for the liver and kidney teams. Two hours later, when it was time to remove the organs, the heart and lungs would come out first. But before any organs were removed, the liver and kidney surgeons had a great deal of work to do — cutting tissues and freeing up blood vessels.

While the others worked, the team from Yale watched and waited. There were risks here, too; the donor might lose blood or become unstable. He might develop an irregular heartbeat. His arterial blood gases could start dropping. Throughout the process, Gail kept Dr. Baldwin up to date on the donor's status.

While the Yale team was waiting, one of the hospital nurses asked Gail who would be receiving the donor's heart and lungs. Gail replied that they were going to a forty-eight-year-old woman with primary pulmonary hypertension, that she was a dancer, and a single mother with a daughter in high school. Invariably, somebody in the operating room inquires about the recipient, and Gail believes strongly in answering that question. In many cases, the doctors and nurses in the OR have recently been through a painful, losing battle to save the donor's life. Often, they have spent the previous day trying to console the grief-stricken family. Although it's too late to help the donor, a second dramatic battle is now in progress. These people have been asked to work all night to save the lives of patients whom they will never meet, and it's only right, Gail feels, to describe the recipient in real terms so the doctors and nurses can feel more connected to this long and difficult process. When the transplant is over, the team at the donor's hospital will be told how the story ended. Even if it ended badly.

Finally, the order was given: "Aorta cross clamp." The aorta was clamped, which completely stopped the donor's circulation. Now the ischemic clock began ticking. Using scissors, sutures, and clamps, the two surgeons swiftly freed up the heart and lungs, but without severing the connections between them. Dr. Hammond picked up the organs and carried them to a back table.

Gently, the surgeons placed the still-connected organs in a metal basin that contained an ice-cold saline solution. They removed as much blood as possible, and inspected the organs again for any anatomical abnormalities that might not have shown up earlier. Then, in an effort to slow down the molecular activity, they cooled the heart and lungs in ice to four degrees Celsius.

Gail picked up the organs and carefully placed them in a sterile plastic bag, where they would be kept cool with saline slush. To further cushion the organs, she inserted this bag into a second one. She then placed the two bags inside a sterile container, which was set in the cooler and packed with ice.

The pilots were already on the runway with special clearance to take off the moment the team arrived. Before the team left the hospital, Gail called Yale to let them know the retrieval had been completed. "We're leaving the O.R.," she told Dr. Baldwin. "We'll see you in an hour and a half."

With Gail carrying the cooler, the team walked briskly to the emergency room, where a waiting ambulance sped them to the airport over deserted country roads. They landed in Connecticut an hour later, just as the sun was rising.

Gail was the last one off the plane. As she turned around to ensure that nothing was left behind, she noticed a bottle of champagne that the pilots had presented to the medical team in honor of Yale's first heart-lung transplant. She grabbed the bottle and carried it off the plane, together with the cooler. The champagne is for Claire, she decided. Except for the fact that Gail hadn't slept all night, this woman with the cooler in one hand and the bottle of champagne in the other looked as if she were going to an early-morning picnic.

Meanwhile, back in the New Haven operating room, I had already been unconscious for several hours. Dr. Baldwin had made a nine-inch incision in my chest, and was preparing to remove my heart and lungs. When the ambulance drove up to the emergency room, Gail picked up the phone and made one last call to Dr. Baldwin. "Begin removal," she said. "We're here." Dr. Baldwin liked to have the donor's organs arrive just as the recipient's old organs were being removed.

As she entered the operating room, Gail was greeted by an astonishing sight: a living, breathing human being, a woman she knew personally, whose chest cavity was not only open, but completely empty. In the space formerly occupied by her heart and lungs, there was nothing at all. "I couldn't believe it," she told me later. "Nobody could. Although we were all wearing masks, I could see the look of amazement on everyone's face. Except for Dr. Baldwin, none of us, not even the surgeons, had ever seen anything like this."

Then, as calmly as if he were putting a child to bed, Dr. Baldwin lowered the new heart and lungs into my chest until they were exactly where he wanted them. This required a little trimming of tissues and vessels, but the organs themselves were untouched. Then he began stitching, first the lungs and then the heart. He connected the pulmonary arteries and sewed the atrium of the new heart to my back atrium wall, which he had left in place.

When all the connections were done, Dr. Baldwin gave the order to "come off bypass." I was gradually taken off the heart-lung machine, which had allowed the surgeons to bypass the blood flow to the heart and lungs. But as often happens, my new heart needed a little assistance in getting started, and Dr. Baldwin called for the electrical paddles. When he applied them my heart jumped, and then started beating on its own. But I was still connected to a respirator, which would remain in place for another day or two.

My new heart and lungs, which had been pale and white because of preservative fluids and a lack of blood, quickly took on a healthy pink glow. When Dr. Baldwin was satisfied that both organs were doing their job, he inserted three large drainage tubes in my chest to remove the excess blood, and attached a wire to my heart in the event that I needed a pacemaker later on. My chest bone was wired shut, and the skin was stapled. As soon as the surgery was over, I was brought directly to the ICU, where I would be stabilized, monitored, and cared for during the next ten days.

The previous night, all but one of my visitors had gone to a nearby hotel to get some sleep. Amara remained in the hospital, where she sat alone in a small waiting area. She dozed off several times during the long night, but every now and then, as a doctor walked by, she was awakened by the sound of a beeper going off. Each time it happened, she had the same nervous response: that this was *her* beeper, which meant that she and I had to leave immediately for Baltimore. Then she'd wake up with a start and remember where she actually was, and what was going on.

Shortly before seven, a nurse told Amara that the organs had arrived from Maine and the transplant was about to begin. A few hours later, somebody else told her that the operation had gone smoothly. Ira had arrived from New Hampshire, and the two of them, exhausted, went out for breakfast.

I knew none of this, of course. While this incredible drama was being played out, I was far away in a remote and mysterious place.

Eight

Humpty Dumpty

FLOATING EFFORTLESSLY in another world, I drifted over to Egypt. I was dressed in white, and next to me was a huge marble column. But why Egypt? Was this a dream? An anesthetically induced hallucination? Was I delirious? Had I died during the transplant and was now entering a different life?

Egypt began to evaporate as I slowly became aware of a buzz of disembodied voices calling my name. "Claire, wake up. It's over, Claire." I awakened gently, feeling no bodily or physical sensation — nothing but pure consciousness and a cacophony of voices, speaking, shouting, proclaiming my name. My name? Why my name? Why weren't they telling me what I wanted to know?

The last thing I had heard was that I might not get the organs. Was the operation successful? Please tell me! Did the transplant happen? *I need to know.* But with the breathing tube in my windpipe, I couldn't speak. Total frustration! Although my hands were tied, I managed to wiggle my fingers in a writing motion. Finally somebody noticed and brought me a pen and paper. I scribbled my question: *Did I get them?*

"Oh, yes," a voice said. "Everything is fine."

Thank you, God! Then back down into the darkness.

Hours later, I awoke in a sweat, flailing around and calling out deliriously. The breathing tube was gone now, and I was having my first heart biopsy. This was the surest way to detect rejection, but so *soon*? The thought of them snipping a piece of my precious new heart, which had just arrived in its new home and hadn't even been given the opportunity to unpack, was so alarming that my heart started racing. My heart was actually running away, or so it seemed. I could see it galloping all over the machines.

Dr. Baldwin rushed in. This heart was still his baby; just this morning he had held it in his hands. I looked up at him and asked for some Valium to calm me down.

"I don't believe in Valium," he said. "I'll give you something better. A mild suppository. You'll love it."

Before I knew it the pellet was inside me, throwing me into a vivid nightmare, except that I wasn't quite sleeping. My head hurt and I struggled to break free. I was trying to scale a high smooth wall with nothing to hold on to.

Half-awake now, I opened my eyes. A blank television monitor stared back from some place above me. To my right, machines ticked away, recording the life inside me through a myriad of tubes. To my left was a door with a windowpane, and now Amara's face was pressed up against the glass. Good! If Amara can see me, I must be alive.

Everyone who entered my room had to suit up: green gown, green mask, green cap, green booties, and latex gloves. They all looked the same, like green blobs; the only way I could tell them apart was to learn to read their eyes. Now a blob with the eyes of my sister came in. For some reason I felt myself winking at her before I passed out again.

I awoke to the rattle of a huge contraption being wheeled in by another green blob. The machine was on top of me, although

I felt nothing. "We're going to take a chest X-ray," said the blob. "We'll be doing this every four hours." Every four hours? Really? They're taking this rather seriously!

An EKG rolled in with a nurse in its wake. Its tentacles attached themselves to me and read the rhythm of my heart. But could it possibly detect how frightened I was? So many questions! How long would this new heart keep beating? How long would these new lungs keep breathing? Would I reject these organs? Would they reject me? What *was* this rejection I'd heard so much about? What form did it take?

I had my own ideas about that. I envisioned the new heart breaking free of its stitches and popping right out of my body. I even wondered whether Dr. Baldwin had sewn it in right. I could swear it was beating deeper in my chest than my old heart did, because I could feel it beating against the bed behind me.

"It's just your imagination," a nurse assured me. "Nothing has changed."

But I knew my body, and something was different. When I asked Dr. Baldwin, he explained that to fit the new heart in, he'd had to position it farther back than the old one. It was nice to know I still had some connection to reality.

As the hours passed, my anxieties increased. Maybe all the fears I had pushed away before the operation were catching up to me now, with a few new ones thrown in. I had been told, for example, that I wouldn't be able to cough after the transplant, that some of my nerves would be severed and I wouldn't feel the familiar coughing reflex. But I was coughing quite a bit, which made me wonder: Did they really know what they were talking about, or were they just pretending so I wouldn't be alarmed?

Maybe they, too, were afraid. Although an endless procession of identical green blobs passed through my isolation, none of them would touch me. I concluded from this that if I were touched, rejection would occur immediately. Rejection, isolation — these were ugly words, and so were the other terms I kept hearing: Biopsy. Necrosis. Transfusion.

Through the glass, I spotted the unmistakable contour of Bernie Siegel's shiny head. I had remembered that he was at Yale, and although we had never met, shortly after the surgery, as soon as I was coherent and able to pick up the phone, I had called him in the hope that he would visit me. I knew him from public television, and had been inspired by his book, *Love, Medicine, and Miracles*. In the book, he wrote in support of the active, questioning, *participating* patient, who must be prepared, if necessary, to tolerate a certain amount of disagreement or even conflict with her doctor.

Although Bernie, too, was covered in green, his gregarious spirit shone through. His bald head was covered by a green cap, but there was no mistaking those twinkling eyes. During his brief visit, Bernie pointed out that when you're in isolation, it can be comforting and therapeutic to see at least a glimpse of the natural world. There was, I remembered, a window behind my bed, with a view of a tree and the sky. But in typical hospital fashion, I was facing the other way, toward the television. As soon as Bernie left, I asked the nurses to turn me around.

On his way out, Bernie came over to give me a hug. I instinctively recoiled: Wouldn't this kick me into instant rejection? But I trusted this man, and I was dying for some human contact. Bernie's hug was wonderful and warm. I took a deep breath, waited a moment — and didn't die. The melting process had begun.

For the first couple of days after surgery, I had been frozen, as if in a block of ice. Maybe God planned it that way as a form of protection: if we express strong emotions too soon after surgery, the stitches could break. But now, for better and for worse, my feelings were starting to return.

On the third day after the operation, two green blobs wheeled in an exercise bicycle. Hold on, I thought. Aren't we rushing things here? I was still on morphine, and just out of major surgery! But Dr. Baldwin wanted me to ride for at least a few minutes, and to my amazement, I did. What a marvelous feeling to be moving my legs again!

With all my fears, I was grateful just to be alive. I was also deeply thankful that a family I had never met had made it possible for me to bypass death and rejoin the world. It was a humbling thought, and I wanted to be worthy of their amazing gift. When I told Gail how I felt, she suggested that I write to the donor's family to express my gratitude. While I couldn't know their identity or sign my name, one of the nurses had told me that my donor was an eighteen-year-old boy from Maine who was killed in a motorcycle accident. And even without names, I could still write to the family from my heart, as it were, and Gail would forward the letter. I did write — once from the hospital, and several more times from home. But during the first weeks after my transplant I was focused more on the gift than on the giver.

I learned later that some transplant recipients feel terribly guilty after the operation because somebody had to die in order for them to live. In the midst of their deep and complicated feelings, they sometimes lose sight of the fact that the donor's death was unrelated to their own prayers or wishes. While I was a beneficiary of my donor's death, I didn't feel responsible for it. I was sad that a young man had died, and I saw myself as a privileged guardian who had been entrusted with a special responsibility. I was living with borrowed organs — not literally borrowed, of course, but that's how it felt. And like everything borrowed, they deserved special care.

Because this was the first heart-lung transplant in New England, the event had generated a fair amount of attention on television and in the papers. Total strangers were sending me cards and letters at the hospital, congratulating me on the transplant and wishing me a long life. And now, on the third day after the transplant, two reporters came in to interview me. The timing was excellent: I was still exhilarated from being able to exercise. When my guests arrived I was all dressed up in yellow silk pajamas and a pink silk bathrobe, a gift from Marilyn. I was so delighted to be moving again that I clowned around and climbed up on the bike, where I posed for a picture with a paper cup on my head.

"Now that the operation is over," one of the reporters asked, "what do you look forward to doing?"

"Regular things," I replied. "I rode this bike today, and it felt wonderful to be able to exercise. When I'm well enough, I'd love to go biking with my daughter. I look forward to some of the simple things that she and I used to take for granted, like walking on the beach together, skating, going to the theater — all the things I've been too sick to do."

"Claire, now that you've had this miracle, what do you want more than anything else?"

"Actually," I said, "I'm dying for a beer right now."

As soon as those words came out of my mouth, I wished I could pull them back in. I was mortified that I had answered this sincere question with such a flippant response. I was also surprised, because I didn't even *like* beer. At least I never had before. But the craving I felt at that moment was specifically for the taste of beer. For some bizarre reason, I was convinced that nothing else in the world could quench my thirst.

That evening, after the reporters had left, an odd notion occurred to me: maybe the donor of my new organs, this young man from Maine, had been a beer drinker. Was it possible, I wondered, that my new heart had reached me with its own set of tastes and preferences? It was a fascinating idea, and for a moment or two I rolled it around in my mind.

Then I let it go. During those early days I had no idea that I would look back on this curious comment as the first of many mysteries after the transplant, or that in the months ahead I would sometimes wonder exactly who was choreographing all these changes in my preferences and my personality.

Was it me, or was it my heart?

What a week! On the fifth day, just two days after I was clowning around with the reporters, I fell into a profound despair, a pit so dark I was afraid I might never find my way out. I had been through the whole cycle — the long wait, the acceptance of death, the miracle of the transplant, and the first indications that my strength and stamina were returning. But now, ironically, a depression settled in so deeply that I didn't think I could make it. Suddenly, being in the ICU was devastating and bewildering. I didn't know who I was or what I was doing here.

My body, the nurses assured me, was doing fine. My recovery was on target, progressing as expected. But it wasn't my body that concerned me. It was everything else.

To start with, I was overwhelmed by these immense and sudden transitions. After months of being housebound, incapacitated, and connected to oxygen tanks, I had been rushed to New Haven for a dangerous operation. I had not only survived, but three days later, just as Gail had promised, I was actually riding an exercise bike with the help of somebody else's lungs and heart. Almost overnight I had gone from total incapacitation to fully functioning. The physical changes alone were so enormous and so abrupt that the rest of me — my mind, my emotions, my soul — hadn't yet caught up. When you awaken from a nightmare, you can shake it off. But it's a lot harder when your nightmare has gone on for years.

Part of what I was experiencing, I now realize, was a postoperative depression that is common among heart surgery and transplant patients. I wish I had known about this at the time, but nobody at the hospital mentioned it. This depression, which typically begins in the ICU within days of the operation, can demoralize even the most optimistic soul. And perhaps my despair reflected the flip side of my unexpected serenity on the eve of the transplant. "It is not uncommon," writes a psychiatrist who has studied patients undergoing heart surgery, "for a person to feel calm while going through what he experiences as a life-endangering situation. . . . When the danger has passed, however, it is usual for a wave of anxiety to sweep over the participant."* He could have been talking about me.

But this was only part of it. In addition to everything else, I was also going through the early stages of an identity crisis. One reason it may have been so severe in my case is that as a dancer, I have always been deeply aware of my body. And now, certain parts of that body — big, major, important parts — had been taken away and replaced with somebody else's. What did that *mean*? Who was this "else"? And how did he, or it, fit into me? I had always known who I was, but who was I *now*? I had

* Richard S. Blacher, "Heart Surgery: The Patient's Experience," in R. S. Blacher (ed.), *The Psychological Experience of Surgery* (New York, 1987), pp. 44–61, p. 47.

been ripped in two and sewn back up, but something was different.

I felt like Humpty Dumpty. I too had experienced a great fall, a traumatic breaking apart. And in my case as well, all the king's horses and all the king's men couldn't put Humpty together again. All the king's horses were the machines that surrounded and monitored me in the ICU; all the king's men were the surgeons and nurses. They were nimble and skilled, and they really did put somebody back together again. But that new, reconstructed person just wasn't me.

Although I couldn't yet put this idea into words, I now believe that what made me so confused and disoriented during my early days in the ICU were the first stirrings of another presence inside me. Increasingly in the months ahead, I would have the feeling that some aspects of my donor's spirit or personality existed within me. During that first week, I knew only that the very center of my being was not fully mine, that it functioned and pulsated with its own rhythm, and a sense of separateness and independence. I didn't understand what was happening to me — but whatever it was, I found it enormously upsetting.

I tried every technique I could think of to get myself back on track. Meditation. Visualization. Affirmations. But nothing worked. I called Gail and told her I felt doomed, that I couldn't go on. Gail was very concerned. She called Barbara Katz, but this time even Barbara wasn't able to help me. I was losing the will to live.

I felt claustrophobic, as if I were trapped and immobilized in an environment that was caving in on me. I'd had the same feeling when I was pregnant with Amara. Although I was thrilled to be having a baby, there was something strange and unknowable about this indeterminate being inside of me that I couldn't control. This mysterious new entity, this future baby, was so precious and vulnerable that the only thing I could do was to take wonderful care of it, which meant taking wonderful care of myself. After the transplant, I had a similar feeling about my new heart and lungs: that they were foreign and beyond my control, but terribly precious and vulnerable.

The dreams I'd had shortly before the transplant, about babies and pregnancy, now took on an additional layer of meaning. My new organs had something in common with a pregnancy that I was just beginning to understand: like a fetus, they constituted a new life force within me, whose parameters were still unclear. No wonder I felt crowded!

Dr. Baldwin appeared in the middle of my depression, as he had been doing at all hours of the day and night ever since the transplant. I couldn't believe it: if I sneezed at three in the morning, he would suddenly materialize to say "Bless you." If I awoke from a dream, he was there. It was almost as if he, too, was living in the hospital. Then one of the nurses told me that in fact he was. For a week after my transplant, he slept in his office with his clothes strewn around and didn't leave the building.

What a relief it was to see him now! While I had long ago stopped feeling awe and reverence toward doctors, in Dr. Baldwin's case I made an exception. Ever since performing this miracle, he had seemed infallible and almost God-like to me. And now, as I looked up at him, I felt certain that with all of his experience, he could help me. The nurses had called me a pioneer, a real bionic woman. I had a zip-locked chest with an implanted heart and lungs. But I also had a mind spinning with confusion.

"Dr. Baldwin, you've taken care of my chest. Would you send in a psychologist to take care of my head?"

"I don't believe in psychologists," he replied. This was a shock. Not believing in Valium I could understand, but psychologists? He and I seemed to be on two different tracks. My feelings, it appeared, were of no real concern to him. Only my physical body was real.

"Just keep riding your bike," Dr. Baldwin said. "Don't even think about your head. Act normal."

"But for me it *is* normal to think about my head!"

"Listen, Claire. Stop all this touchy-feely stuff and get on with your life. You came to *me* for this radical procedure, not Bernie Siegel."

I felt shattered when he said that. I believed, and still do, that the practice of medicine depends on both the Baldwins *and* the Siegels, and I expect that in the not-too-distant future, physicians and healers will find ways to combine and integrate these two approaches. But while we seem to be moving in that direction, new attitudes take time. For the moment, I was a patient in this hospital where Dr. Baldwin was in charge. And now my enormous gratitude toward this man was mixed with feelings of betrayal. Although he had performed this difficult operation, and had done it brilliantly, he seemed to have no idea what it felt like to be on the receiving end. What troubled me even more was that he didn't seem interested in finding out.

In retrospect, I was being unrealistic to expect Dr. Baldwin to help me emotionally. We all see the world through our own eyes, and while Dr. Baldwin's vision seemed limited to me, he was a well-regarded surgeon who had alleviated a great deal of suffering for hundreds of people. And for all my frustration that he didn't have the sensitivities and concerns of Bernie Siegel, Dr. Baldwin had saved my life.

When he left the room, I obediently climbed up on the bike and pedaled like crazy.

"Just act normal," the doctor had said. But what was "normal"? I wasn't normal before, and I certainly wasn't normal now.

Often, when I'm depressed, the worse I feel, the more creative I become. Sitting on the bike, I resolved that as soon as I was strong enough, I would start a support group for transplant recipients. Although this hospital had been performing heart transplants for years, there was no place for these patients to talk to each other. Who else could possibly understand what this operation was like, and all the things it meant?

The workout took the edge off my anger, but I still ached with confusion. Being thrust back into life, being reborn after being so close to death — this was overwhelming. It would have been easier — not better, necessarily, but easier and more natural, if I had simply let go. One reason I had been ambivalent about this operation was that assuming it worked, it would mean dying twice. After a transplant you're thrown back into life with the knowledge that some day you'll have to go through the whole process of dying all over again.

Rationally, I knew that my new life was almost surely a blessing, even if it didn't yet feel that way. But emotionally, being reborn was painful and terribly difficult — just as being born must be for an infant leaving the womb and being slapped into its first breath. The physical reality of a transplant was so immense that even I, who spent so much of my life in the world of feelings, hadn't been able to see past the medical facts to even imagine the enormous emotional ramifications. I wished somebody had warned me that these issues might come up.

A day or so later I awoke up from a nap to find a man I had never seen before, who appeared to be in his mid-thirties, sitting across from me. He introduced himself as Gary Thorpe, and he told me that five years earlier he had undergone a heart transplant at this same hospital. When he returned for his periodic checkups, Gail would ask him to talk with some of the newer patients, just as she would later ask me to do the same. Gary seemed to understand what I was feeling, and his presence in my room was enormously meaningful and comforting — for the simple reason that he was alive and talking to me. Although this man was a total stranger, I suddenly felt closer to him than to anyone else on this planet. He knew what I knew.

Within minutes a surge of hope was moving through me. Gary knew exactly what it felt like to have your heart pulled out of your body and replaced by the heart of a stranger. And not just any stranger, but somebody whose involuntary and unchosen death had given you life.

"What was it like when you got out of here?" I asked him. I couldn't imagine how I would possibly cope when it came time to leave the hospital. I could barely imagine leaving the ICU, where, for all my recent unhappiness, I felt safe and protected. The doctors and nurses were always looking in on me. Maybe that's why they called it the ICU. I see you! How could I ever survive outside the womb?

"You just take it day by day," Gary said. "Very slowly at first, but it gets better all the time. You'll see."

After Gary Thorpe's visit, my depression lifted. As soon as he left, I again thought about a support group. I was so grateful to this man that I wanted to give others what he had given me. There was, after all, a growing community of people who were having heart or heart-lung transplants, and we obviously needed each other. Spiritually and emotionally, nobody else could truly understand us.

Now I had even more reason to be thankful. Right after the surgery, Dr. Baldwin sent my old heart and lungs over to pathology, where one of the doctors estimated that my lungs had suffered so much damage that if it hadn't been for the transplant, I would have been dead within a month. My heart was even worse; the right side was in total failure. It's a good thing Gail had summoned me in May; June might have been too late.

At the time, I didn't fully understand that a transplant involves a simultaneous adjustment to two major changes: the loss of your own vital organs, and the concurrent acceptance of new ones. And in case these changes aren't complicated enough, they can only occur when a life is lost — a life the recipient knows little or nothing about, except that a piece of it was transferred to her own body to give her life. These are enormous issues, and although the operation is over in a matter of hours, an introspective recipient could spend years trying to deal with all the ramifications of the transplant.

And what about those missing organs? As diseased as they were, my old heart and lungs were a part of me. We knew each other like old friends. Although they had caused me pain and suffering, we had been through a lot together. I read somewhere that when sick people are given a theoretical choice among different illnesses, most of them prefer their own. Your illness may not be pleasant, but at least it's yours. It's familiar, and you know how to cope with it. It's not that I seriously missed my old heart and lungs — or my old illness, for that matter. But getting used to not having them was harder than I expected.

It also took longer. Years after the transplant, I was walking down the street one evening when the thought occurred to me that for forty-seven years my life had revolved around the fact that my heart was defective. I had danced anyway, but even so, much of my activity and my identity, especially during childhood, had centered on my heart murmur. Suddenly I remembered: I don't have that heart murmur anymore. Only then did it hit me with full force: I don't even have that *heart* anymore.

All my life I had watched the pained and contorted faces of the many doctors who listened to my old heart with their stethoscopes. I always wondered: What are they hearing? How bad is it? Now, after the transplant, I had the strange and liberating experience of watching doctors listen to my heart without a frown. In the hospital, some of them would actually smile.

Toward the end of my stay in the ICU, Ira called from New Hampshire to say that he was driving down for another visit. A few minutes later, a nurse came in to say that my ex-husband was in the waiting room.

"That's impossible," I said. "I just spoke to him, and he won't arrive until tonight."

"I don't know, Claire. He's out there, and he says he's your ex-husband."

As I was trying to imagine who this could possibly be, David, my *second* ex-husband, came into the room.

For all I knew, when you woke up with someone else's heart in your body, forgetting an ex-husband or two wasn't all that unusual. Maybe it happens to everyone. It's a good thing there are only two of them, I thought. At least I *think* there are only two. In my current state, anything seemed possible.

When David walked in, my heart was actually palpitating. We had been out of touch for years, following our bitter divorce. Seeing him, I felt a sudden rush of mixed memories — the arguments and the hurt, but also the love and the passion. His showing up here was the first emotional shock to hit my heart since the transplant, and I started to worry that it might lead to rejection.

Then I realized that I was actually *feeling* with my new heart. This heart, which less than a week ago was beating in another person's body, was now feeling my feelings. And it seemed to be feeling them more powerfully than my own heart had, at least in recent months. Maybe this new heart could withstand more emotion. Maybe it was more resilient. Maybe my old heart could no longer contain sharp, intense feelings. In recent months my emotions had become faded and washed out, less red-blooded, more ethereal, and spiritualized.

It was hard work, getting used to this new me.

Nine

Stayin' Alive

THREE AND A HALF weeks after the transplant, Dr. Baldwin determined that I was ready to leave the hospital and move into a condominium a few miles away. This, of course, was a dramatic, tangible sign that I was no longer in any immediate danger. But once again my emotions lagged behind the rapid pace of my physical recovery. For all my ambivalence about hospital life, I was terrified at the prospect of leaving this high-tech sanctuary — my new haven, so to speak — and venturing out into the dangerous world of potential infection. I imagined an army of hostile germs who were well trained and heavily armed. They were lying in wait just outside the hospital walls, preparing to launch a murderous assault on my immune-suppressed body.

And if the germs didn't get me, there were other, more basic perils to worry about. Would my new heart continue beating, or would rejection set in the moment I left the building? Would my lungs continue to function, or had they been protected since the transplant by some invisible, magic hospital shield whose power would dissipate as soon as I stepped outside?

Despite these fears, I was increasingly optimistic about the future. As the days passed, I had become progressively stronger.

My gait became steadier and more confident, and every day I walked a little farther in the hospital corridors. For the first time in ages, my nails took on a fresh pink coloring.

But when I took my first shower and accidentally dropped the soap, I experienced a moment of real panic. Parts of me were still functioning on my old, pretransplant operating system, and I knew from bitter experience that if I bent down to pick up the soap, I might be risking a bad attack of angina. I was about to leave the soap on the floor when I realized that this was a left-over fear from my previous life. When I scooped it up with no ill effects, I felt a rush of surprise and jubilation. Another victory! Day by day, just as Gary Thorpe had promised.

My mood was improving, too. Ever since I had arrived in New Haven, just about every conversation, every question, answer, and comment had been understandably serious and important. Now, as my strength increased, so did my hopes. Given a taste of health, I longed to laugh and have some fun. My spirit was returning!

Looking ahead to my release from the hospital, Amara had been reading through a list of do's and don'ts for recovering heart transplant recipients. "Mom," she informed me, "you can have sex in about six weeks, about the time you can start driving again." I burst out laughing — not only at the linking of these disparate activities, but also because for years, every time I had tried to talk to Amara about sex, she became mortified and immediately changed the subject. But she seemed to have no hesitation about discussing *my* sex life. Now it was Mom's turn to be embarrassed.

On my final day at Yale, the hospital officials arranged a press conference to discuss my transplant. When Gail asked me to say a few words about my experience, I was thrilled. She came to my room to collect me, and laughingly shook her head. "Claire,

would you fix your hair, please? You look like a porcupine!"
Now that I was rejoining the world, here was another big ad-
justment: I would once again be responsible for my appearance.
Simply being alive was no longer enough.

At the press conference, which was held in a crowded conference room, I expressed my deep and sincere appreciation to
the medical staff. When Dr. Baldwin described how well I was
doing, I felt enormously proud. His comments took on an additional weight in this public setting, and between his positive
projections and the attentive gaze of the audience, I began to
feel more confident about leaving the hospital. As he spoke, I
looked down at my pink, healthy nails and resolved never to
wear nail polish again — a promise I soon broke.

I was surprised to hear Dr. Baldwin describe my recovery as
"unremarkable." At first I thought he was kidding, until I realized that he was referring only to the physical aspects of my recuperation, which had indeed gone smoothly. But I wondered
how a doctor could so easily separate a person's body from the
rest of her being.

When the press conference was over there was a farewell re-
ception in my honor, where Gail discreetly gave me a sip of the
champagne she had removed from the plane on the morning of
the operation. When all the goodbyes were said and all my tears
were cried, she wheeled me outside — my first moment out of
doors since Bob, Barbara, and Amara had rushed me to the hospital. Back then, on the final afternoon of my previous life, the
skies were darkened by rain clouds and illuminated by a rainbow. Today, fittingly, the sun was so bright I had to squint.
Slowly and deliberately, I inhaled a deep breath of fresh air into
my new lungs. It hurt a little, but this was a pain I was happy to
feel.

*   *   *

The condominium I was moving into would function as a kind of medical halfway house; I would stay there for about three months, returning to the hospital for weekly checkups. I would be sharing the apartment with a live-in housekeeper, and for the first three weeks I would also have round-the-clock nursing care.*

During my summer in the condo, I had the oddly exotic experience of living a more or less normal life, without oxygen, pain, or major worries. There were a few minor restrictions: to minimize the risk of infection, for example, I was told to stay away from animals and avoid going into crowds.

These limitations seemed even less restrictive in view of the bold and generous new freedoms I could now enjoy. For the first time in ages, I could eat almost anything I wanted: "Order a pizza if you like," the doctor had said. Amazing! I had expected a million dietary prohibitions after the transplant, and I was prepared to obey them all. But compared to being sick, this was — well, a piece of cake.

Being able to eat freely was such a joyous change in my routine that at first I could hardly believe it. I stuck mostly to fruit, grains, and vegetables, but shortly after leaving the hospital I treated myself to a hamburger in a restaurant, which came gar-

---

* I was extremely fortunate to have all of my transplant-related expenses covered by the Massachusetts Transplant Fund, a charitable endowment that was established in the mid-1980s through voluntary "checkoff" contributions from taxpayers on their state tax forms. The fund was authorized to reimburse Massachusetts residents for "any and all expenses related to a medically necessary transplant," and because I was one of the first recipients to apply for help, the subsidies were very generous. What my insurance company didn't cover, the Transplant Fund did.

nished with an olive on a toothpick. The hamburger was exciting enough, but what I really craved was that little green olive! I was so accustomed to avoiding salty foods that my initial instinct was to push it away. But I love olives, and I must have stared at this one a good five minutes before I finally surrendered. I half expected the earth to open up and devour me, but nothing happened. Freedom!

Now I could eat like a regular person — even if that person wasn't quite me. To my surprise, I developed a sudden fondness for certain foods I hadn't liked before. I had always enjoyed sweets, but now I was eating a lot more of them — especially Snickers Bars and Reese's Peanut Butter Cups.

I was also showing a strange new affinity for green peppers, which I had never liked and had always removed from my salads. After the transplant I found myself adding green peppers to every conceivable dish, although I had no idea why.

And when I was finally allowed to drive again, my car practically steered itself to the nearest Kentucky Fried Chicken. This made no sense at all, because I never go to fast-food outlets. But for some inexplicable reason, I felt a craving for chicken nuggets. Like my earlier yearning for beer, this sudden desire for chicken would be explained only later.

In the condominium, I quickly settled into a comfortable daily routine. While Dot, my housekeeper, prepared breakfast, I started the morning with yoga, meditation, and twenty minutes on the bike. During the day I'd walk around the neighborhood, talk on the phone, read a book, or go shopping with Dot. I was a little embarrassed at how quickly I grew accustomed to having a full-time housekeeper, and how easily this luxury came to feel like a necessity. Before I knew it, I was relying on Dot so completely that I almost forgot how, as recently as a month ago, I had managed to survive with very little help, even on days when I could barely stand up.

Within a couple of weeks, I started a support group for transplant recipients. Gail was enormously helpful, especially when it came to recruiting people who had either undergone heart or heart-lung transplants, or were waiting for one. About sixteen people attended the initial meeting at my condo. All of us were happy and relieved to discover that we were not alone, that other people in our situation faced some of the same problems we did. I was especially pleased that after years of receiving help from family, friends, and medical professionals, I was finally able to give something back.

The support group grew quickly, and before long we split into three smaller sections: one for recipients; a second section for those who were waiting for transplants; and a third group for family members and close friends of the people in the other two groups. By this time I had moved back to Boston, but I continued attending and leading the monthly meetings. I even took a course on how to lead a support group, and shared my new knowledge with other volunteer leaders.

While I looked forward to these meetings, they were usually accompanied by a certain amount of sadness. Almost every time we met, there would be news of yet another friend or acquaintance from the transplant program who had died since our last meeting. Sometimes the cause was post-transplant rejection, but more often we heard about somebody who had been waiting months for a transplant, and whose heart finally gave out before a suitable donor could be found. As we were well aware, there are never enough organ donors for all the people who need them.

When a patient died, the doctors and the hospital staff tried to protect us from knowing about it. They asked us to help newer patients by visiting them in the ICU, but when one of these patients died, they kept it secret. We resented this terribly. We knew perfectly well that all of us, whether pretransplant or post, were living on borrowed time.

One of my regular visitors at the condo was the new man in my life. Kal was a Boston psychologist whom I had known and liked before the transplant, and now that I was feeling stronger, our relationship started heating up. But despite Amara's reminder that sex was permissible six weeks after the operation, the prospect of being intimate with Kal frightened me — in much the same way, I suppose, that men who have undergone a heart attack or bypass surgery are often afraid that resuming sexual activity will land them back in the hospital, or worse. I could just imagine myself having to stop in the middle of a passionate embrace to say, "Excuse me, but I think my heart is rejecting!" It didn't sound very romantic.

My apprehensions about sex didn't mean I wasn't interested. Now that I was feeling more human and less like a robot, erotic thoughts and feelings had once again begun to stir within me. And I was definitely interested in Kal. I just wasn't sure I was ready for this next stage, and I didn't want to push my luck. I was so sick before the transplant it was hard to believe I could go back to being a normal, active adult without having to sacrifice at least one important pleasure in return for my newfound health.

One day, as Kal was driving up to see me, a strange question crept into my mind. Although I hadn't thought much about my donor, I was acutely aware that I was now living with a man's heart. And I wondered: Is it conceivable that this male heart might affect me sexually? Probably not, but who knew for sure?

My new heart did seem to be affecting my personality. I noticed that I no longer felt lonely, even when I was by myself. On weekdays, when I was separated from Amara and my friends, I didn't miss them much. Sometimes I had the feeling that somebody else was in there with me, that in some intangible way, my sense of "I" had become a kind of "we." Although I couldn't always detect this extra presence, at times it almost felt as if a second soul were sharing my body. I wondered about these feelings, but I still wasn't ready to take them seriously. Because they didn't fit into any category I was aware of, I dismissed them.

But this new male energy did seem to be affecting me. Until the transplant, I had spent most of my adult life either in a relationship with a man or hoping to be in one. But for years after the operation, while I still felt attracted to men, I didn't feel that same need to have a boyfriend. I was freer and more independent than before, as if I had taken on a more masculine outlook. Most men — at least the ones I've known — just don't crave the closeness of an intimate connection the way women do. They may enjoy being in a relationship, but they don't feel incomplete without one. For the first time in my life, I didn't either.

It took years after the transplant before I was finally in an extended relationship with a man. I was still meeting men and enjoying their company, but generally, as we grew closer, something in me seemed to be pushing these men away. I occasionally wondered if my male heart might be jealous, as if this presence I was feeling was reluctant to share me with anyone else.

My personality was changing, too, and becoming more masculine. I was more aggressive and more assertive than I used to be, and more confident as well. I felt I knew things that men knew, things I hadn't known as a woman and that seemed to have come to me from some other place. It was a subtle feeling, as though I'd been entrusted with some secret knowledge that I didn't completely understand.

Even my walk became more masculine. "Mom," said Amara, "why are you walking like that? You're kind of lumbering, like a football player." Then a dance friend said, "Claire, you're really strutting." It was, I realized, the stride of a virile young male, the kind of strut that John Travolta used in *Saturday Night Fever,* with that swaggering self-assurance and that smile, walking in rhythm with everybody stopping in their tracks to watch this youthful, vital man coming down the street. Then I remembered that the theme song of that movie was, appropriately enough, "Stayin' Alive."

Whatever was going on with this new masculine energy, it wasn't limited to my walk. Or perhaps my new walk was a metaphor for the way I now was moving through the world without feeling restricted. I felt a new power that I associated with masculinity, strength, and vibrancy. A certain feminine tentativeness had fallen away, and was replaced by a new confidence.

Years after the operation, my cousin Sharon said that when she first hugged me after the transplant, I felt different from before. "You were giving off heat," she said. "Like the heat you sometimes feel when you hug a man."

Sometimes people ask me whether my sexual preferences have changed since the transplant. While this hasn't happened in any overt way, I am often drawn to women whom I, as a woman, don't feel are especially attractive. The women whose looks I liked before the transplant tended to be tall, slender, and dark, but after the transplant I also found myself looking at women who are shorter, rounder, and blonder — as if some male energy within me were responding to them.

And while I've always been a confirmed heterosexual, after the transplant, at a conference in Boston, I became friendly with a beautiful blond Dutch woman. We spent time together, and when the conference was over I invited her to stay at my place for a couple of days. It was all very innocent on my part, or so I thought, but as soon as we were alone she made it clear in several suggestive ways that she was interested in a sexual relationship. I declined her invitation, but her surprise at my lack of interest made me wonder what kinds of signals I had been sending out without realizing it. I also had several dreams in which I was living with, or getting married to, a woman. These images puzzled me, and in the dreams I often asked: Why am I with a woman when *I'm* a woman? Shouldn't my partner be a man? But these questions were never answered.

As for Kal, our first time together after the transplant went rather well, despite my awkwardness. I was nervous and excited, and there was a fair amount of starting and stopping as I felt my heart beating faster than I was accustomed to. But Kal was right there with me, encouraging and reassuring me. He had always been kind and considerate, and before the transplant, during some of the worst days of my illness, he had come to my house to bathe my chilly hands and feet with warm water, or to cook me an occasional meal. More than any man I've known, Kal was a caretaker.

During my recuperation, it looked as if he and I might have a future together. But as soon as I moved back to Boston, he ended the relationship. He said he just wasn't capable of making a long-term commitment, and while that may have been true, I believe there was more to it. Some people, and Kal was one of them, are fulfilled only when they're caring for someone who needs them in certain basic ways. As soon as I was healthy again, Kal could no longer play that role.

I was terribly sad when Kal left, and I wondered: Am I *ever* going to get this right? Alan had wanted me as long as I was healthy; Kal had been with me as long as I wasn't. Somewhere, I told myself, there's a man who will love me in sickness and in health. And while I didn't need that man in the same pressing way I used to, it would still be awfully nice if he turned up.

In the early fall, just before I returned home to Massachusetts, a woman I had met at the hospital invited me to join her in temple on Rosh Hashanah, the Jewish New Year. Sitting in the service, so many emotions filled me and found their way through my body to my tearing eyes. I missed Amara, who was now back in school after the summer break. I thought of my mother, whose *Yahrzeit* — the anniversary of her death — was the previous day. And I was filled with bittersweet memories of gains and losses. I never thought I'd be here today to remember it all.

What would this new year bring? In Jewish tradition, Rosh Hashanah marks the season when God decides who will live and who will die. Given my recent history, it was incredible to think that exactly a year ago, I, of all people, had been inscribed in the Book of Life. Apparently God had wanted me to live. And while I didn't want to be presumptuous, I hoped that after everything I had just been through, He would extend my lease a few more years.

That morning I had put on a dress with my scar showing above the neckline. The transplant scar was a long vertical line down my upper body, and when it reached my stomach it intersected with another scar from the three enormous drainage tubes that Dr. Baldwin had put in my chest at the end of the operation. There I was, sitting in synagogue with a huge cross engraved on my body.

I was proud of my scars, and I wore them like a war wound. I was grateful to be alive, and especially grateful to be here, in this service, where I could feel and express my appreciation for being alive. I knew that in the future, my scar would serve as a kind of balance, a reminder of those difficult and painful years of illness. It was still a little hard to believe, but it seemed reasonable to hope that those times might be gone forever.

Shortly after I left the condominium and moved back home, I had the most unforgettable dream of my life. In this dream, which I described at the beginning of my story,

> *I'm in an open, outdoor place with grass all around. It's summer. With me is a young man who is tall, thin, and wiry, with sandy-colored hair. His name is Tim — I think it's Tim Leighton, but I'm not sure. I think of him as Tim L. We're in a playful relationship, and we're good friends.*
>
> *It's time for me to leave, to join a performing group of acrobats. I start to walk away from him, but I suddenly feel that something remains unfinished between us. I turn around and go back to him to say goodbye. Tim is standing there watching me, and he seems happy when I return.*
>
> *Then we kiss. And as we kiss, I inhale him into me. It feels like the deepest breath I've ever taken, and I know that Tim will be with me forever.*

I awoke from this dream absolutely exhilarated. When I breathed Tim into me, it was as if I had breathed in new life. I also felt I had finally integrated the new heart and lungs within me. But even more important, I knew, somehow, that the young man in this dream was my donor. I couldn't prove it, of course. But sometimes you just know, and this was one of those times.

Naturally, I was eager to verify this information. But the transplant program at the hospital observed a strict code of confidentiality, and Yale wasn't unique in that respect. In 1988, every American hospital where organ transplants were done maintained an ironclad rule that the donor's identity could never be revealed to the recipient, and vice versa.

I called Gail anyway. While I knew she couldn't reveal my donor's name, I hoped she would tell me whether the name in my dream was correct. When I described the dream and asked her about Tim L., there was a momentary silence.

"No, you can't know that," she finally said. "I'm not supposed to discuss this with you. Please, Claire, let it go. Even if you succeed in tracking down the family, you would just be opening a can of worms."

"What do you mean?"

"You can never predict how the donor's family will respond. People have all kinds of unexpected reactions. If you're curious about the donor, that's only natural; I would be, too. But please let it go. This whole topic is too emotional and unpredictable."

Although I was terribly disappointed by Gail's response, I agreed to drop the subject. But other dreams, and other changes, soon forced me to reconsider that decision.

Ten

RoboClaire

A FEW WEEKS later, Tim appeared in another dream.

I'm a man who has changed into a woman. I'm driving fast, speeding around a series of hairpin turns and loving it. Suddenly I can't make one of the turns, and I fly across the highway, over the divide and into the oncoming traffic. It's a freeing, wild feeling, like flying in the air, a little like the ending of Thelma and Louise *as the car drives off the cliff. I'm no longer confined by the road, and I feel boundless.*

The next thing I know, I'm with a whole new family. They're preparing for their daughter's wedding, which is tomorrow. Their daughter is young, blond, and attractive. Now I'm a man again, and I tell my new family that I have to leave on my plane to meet a girl who is waiting to marry me back where I came from. Then I realize I shouldn't go to her, that it's not right, that I should stay here.

I'm surrounded by my new family. They describe how they pulled me out of the wreckage after I had crashed. I tell them I'm grateful, that there is nothing to fear in death, and that I remember nothing from the moment I flew off the highway. I

*don't even know whether I died. It's like forgetting a dream af-
ter you wake up.*

I didn't really understand this dream until I realized that the
"I" in the dream wasn't necessarily me. Unlike the inhaling
dream, this one seemed to be taking place not from my perspective, but from Tim's. The fact that "I" was both male and female in the dream seemed to support this idea. As far as I could
remember, I had never had a cross-gender dream before the
transplant. Until now, I had always been a woman.

The dream made more sense when I examined it from the
perspective of my donor. It seemed to be about Tim's decision
to stay on in this strange new world — that is, in my body. He
flew over the dividing line of the highway, but he was also crossing a larger boundary — between life and death, or perhaps between one life and another. Although he felt a strong pull to go
back, he made a conscious decision to stay.

The dream was also about my own ambivalence about staying
in my new world — the same ambivalence that came up during
my severe, post-transplant depression. At the time, I was strug-
gling with whether to give up or to jump back into life with my
new, altered identity. In the dream, I reaffirmed the decision I
had already made in my waking life — to stay alive. And
Tim — or at least the Tim I was imagining in my unconscious
mind — had made a similar choice.

And what was being celebrated in this dream? A marriage,
the union between a man and a woman. This seemed to be a
symbolic reference to the integration of Tim's heart and lungs
into my body and soul. We were joined. Tim was now part of
me, and I was part of him.

The idea that a transplant recipient might have a dream from
the donor's perspective is an intriguing one, and it brings to

mind a story I heard later from another recipient. This man said that he never remembered his dreams, except for this one, which occurred right after his transplant. He dreamed he had died, but that when you die, you don't really die; you just enter somebody else's body. As the dream began, he went into a darkened state, where he saw himself being covered by a sheet. His family and friends came to him, and he knew he had to pray to bring in the light. The room became brighter and brighter until he found himself in a bright, strange place where everything was completely different. He found this experience so frightening that describing it years later still made him anxious. His dream, like mine, seemed to have been experienced from the perspective of the donor's heart, a wandering entity that suddenly found itself in an unfamiliar world.

Which is exactly where I ended up in my waking life — in an unfamiliar world. Four months after the transplant, I finally moved back home. But while I was returning to the same apartment, the same furnishings, and the same friends, I was astonished to find that nothing from my old life was entirely recognizable. The four months I was away seemed more like four decades.

My friends and relatives seemed foreign to me now. I still knew them and loved them, but who on earth were they? It was like attending your thirtieth high school reunion and seeing familiar faces tucked under layers of aging. You recognize these people, but you have no idea who they really are. At the time, I thought it was like having amnesia. But I now believe that I still hadn't figured out who *I* was after the transplant, which made it difficult to reconnect with anybody else.

My bumpy reentry reminded me of the movie *RoboCop*. The main character is a former police officer who, after being shot, is transformed into a robot in whom some remnants of the original person still exist. When RoboCop returns home, he finds the same house and the same people he knew when he was fully human, except that everyone and everything seems slightly off. I had a similar reaction when I came back, including the part about feeling less than fully human.

To some degree I had to reestablish my relationship with every significant person in my life, starting with Amara. She had been loving and attentive while I was dying, but now that I was alive and increasingly well, she and I had some adjustments to make. During my illness, a lot of emotion and anger in our relationship had understandably gone unexpressed, and for a long time I had neither the strength nor the spirit to really engage her. If a problem wasn't easy to resolve, we simply deferred it until some future date — which neither of us ever expected to see.

But that unlikely future had now arrived, which meant that various normal but long-suppressed tensions could finally be expressed. A few days after I returned home, Amara and I had a major blowup — I no longer remember why — and soon we were really yelling at each other. During a particularly heated moment, I caught a glimpse of myself in a mirror. Suddenly our fight didn't matter; all I could think of was *My God, check out this lung power!* I started laughing, and I quickly turned away so Amara wouldn't think I was mocking her.

But when she noticed my reflection in the mirror, Amara started laughing, too.

"Watch out, kid," I said, "because now I can outyell you!"

It was wonderful to be able to fight with her, and to reestablish a more complete relationship with Amara that didn't center around my illness. It was also gratifying to be able to use my voice again, and to express what I was feeling.

Although we had some difficult moments, it was amazing to

see how our relationship matured and solidified after the transplant. Now that I was healthy, Amara once again felt free to criticize me, just as she used to, and to use her dry wit to mock me. My daughter the rationalist especially enjoyed teasing me about meditation, my New Age inclinations, and my tendency to see the world in psychological terms. If I started describing a dream, she would roll her eyes and say, "Here we go again." If I dared to offer a metaphysical comment or a mystical interpretation, she'd come back with, "Why do you say that, O Spiritual One?" Amara has always been less ethereal than I, and funnier, too. She can be cutting without being cruel, and even when the jokes were at Mom's expense — and they usually were — I generally enjoyed them. It was wonderful to see that after all this time, Amara was also getting *her* spirit back.

During my illness, we had both lost touch with our earlier years together, when we were happy and free. As a child, Amara loved to dance with me, but around the time I became sick she stopped dancing and took up sports. Then, in a moving gesture of empathy and identification — although she would never have agreed with that interpretation — she developed asthma and began using an inhaler before, and sometimes even during, her lacrosse games. About a year after the transplant, when it was apparent that my survival was no longer in doubt, Amara no longer needed the inhaler. She also started dancing again. She had even broken up with her boyfriend shortly before the transplant, although she and Danny got back together after the operation. The parallels between our lives were quite remarkable.

It was only in retrospect that I could fully appreciate the enormous and depressing impact that my illness had had on her. Through no fault of her own, Amara had essentially been robbed of her youth. She had longed to be a normal kid without having to worry about a mother who was always in bed with an oxygen tank. As my primary caretaker, Amara had been more concerned with helping me stay alive than with the various emotional and social complexities of being a teenage girl — not to mention a teenage girl in a single-parent household with no siblings and a dying mother. While other kids her age were dealing with the standard adolescent manifestations of identity and rebellion, Amara was learning about bank accounts, writing checks, and paying bills. She was forced to think about questions like, If Mom dies before I finish high school, where will I live?

Now, at the age of sixteen, during this delayed adolescence, it was finally safe for her to separate from me. It was as if my new lungs enabled Amara, too, to breathe easier. She occasionally exploded at me as she slowly began to trust in my strength and my resilience. But if her anger was sometimes loud and intense, so was her love. She hugged me hard, picked me up and whirled me around, dancing and laughing. What a delight for both of us, this new knowledge that I wasn't about to break in two, that I wasn't about to die.

"Thank you for two things, Mom," she told me after the transplant. "Thank you for living, and thank you for trusting me when you were sick."

It wasn't until well after the transplant, when Amara left for college, that she could finally put those terrible times behind her. She went to Colgate University in upstate New York, where, on snowy days, the students would slide down the enormous hills on cafeteria trays. At first she held back, but when she finally tried it, the freedom and the sheer exhilaration of those rides brought a sense of closure to a long and stressful period in her life. Mom was finally healthy, and Amara was finally free.

A few months earlier, at her high school graduation, we had both been in tears. This was the day I had lived for and prayed for, the event I had so fervently hoped I would be able to attend. Sitting in the audience, almost overcome by emotion, I recalled Mary Gohlke's words of encouragement when I had called her shortly after learning that PPH was a fatal disease: she had advised me to set goals for myself, and I had. My long-term goal had been to stay alive until Amara's graduation, and now, incredibly, I had reached it. Knowing that I hadn't reached it alone, I silently gave thanks to God for keeping me alive, sustaining me, and allowing me to reach this glorious moment.

While my relationship with Amara was rich and engaging, the rest of my reentry to civilian life was more tenuous and problematic. I felt like an alien who had just been dropped on this strange and unfamiliar planet. What was I doing here, and where did I fit in? And how could people actually *live* like this? Judging from what I saw on television, human society was even more violent and fragmented than I had remembered. But why? I didn't get it. I've since heard that astronauts sometimes experience a similar kind of bewilderment and incredulity when they return to their home planet and become reacquainted with its shocking and turbulent fury.

I now seemed to feel things more deeply, as if my new heart were indeed capable of more intense emotions. When I was happy, I was often elated; when I was depressed, the pain was severe. I was also more sensitive to other people's suffering. Once, at the supermarket, a checkout clerk cut herself on the edge of a paper bag and I literally felt her pain. "Oh, that must hurt!" I said to her. As I walked away I thought to myself, You've been through a heart-lung transplant and *this* got your attention? But it did.

People have asked me in similar situations, "Why are you so

concerned? That's trivial, after what you've been through." But it's not trivial. The transplant was real, but so is a paper cut. Pain is pain.

For a long time after the transplant I couldn't tolerate violent images or scenes of brutality. The nightly news became unbearable, and movies were often too disturbing to sit through. The first movie I saw in my new life was *The Last Temptation of Christ,* and while I had loved the novel, the film version seemed so brutal that I walked out after a few scenes. Even *A Fish Called Wanda,* a well-made comedy, struck me as so cruel and mean-spirited that I couldn't enjoy it.

It wasn't until *Field of Dreams,* a few months later, that I enjoyed going to the movies again. Judging from the title, it should have been ideal for me — and it was. For one thing, the movie takes dreams seriously, even when they seem far-fetched or difficult to understand. For another, *Field of Dreams* is very respectful toward different forms of reality, including strange or "impossible" events that can't be explained in conventional or scientific ways. Finally, the movie suggests, as I was increasingly coming to believe, that the boundaries between life and death, or between this life and other possible lives, might not be as permanent or as immutable as we generally assume.

The same could be said of the movie *Ghost,* which I saw a few months later and which scared me half to death. *Ghost* tells the story of a good man who is murdered, but whose spirit is temporarily unable to leave this world. Eventually his ghost finds a medium and communicates through her, and at one point even takes over her body. But until then, the ghost's attempts to communicate with the familiar world around him are excruciating. His body, which he still inhabits, is now invisible, but he has acquired new powers, including the ability to pass through walls by leaning into them. That's the image that really got to me, because just a few weeks after the transplant, I'd had a similar experience in a dream.

In this dream I had walked right through a wall. I stood up against it, and gently, very gently, leaned my body in and passed right through to the other side. It was easy and painless, as if my body had no density. I was euphoric when it happened, from having effortlessly passed through a barrier that had always seemed impenetrable — like the boundary between life and death. I was no longer a mere mortal; I had cheated death! After years of seeing myself as weak and incapacitated, I could breathe again, walk again, and even ride a bike. Why *not* walk through walls? All my fears had evaporated. I could do anything!

On awakening from the dream, I immediately thought of the transplant, where I had crossed over briefly to the other side of life and then returned to this world, which now seemed both foreign and familiar. I felt like the ghost had in the movie, before he found the medium: having crossed the boundary, I could no longer relate to the people around me. I didn't know it then, but this theme of crossing over a major divide and then returning would become a common theme in my dreams.

I was alone when I saw *Ghost*. Watching the film's depiction of life on both sides of the hitherto impenetrable wall of death, I felt that I, too, was now living on the other side. I felt ghostlike myself that night, as if I weren't real, as if I had no body. As I got into my car I was shaking. Whose ghost was I? That was easy: the ghost of Tim, the boy who had died. In the dream, and again after watching the movie, I was experiencing the transplant from two different perspectives: that of the living recipient, and that of the deceased donor.

When I arrived home from *Ghost* I was crying hysterically.

Fortunately, Amara was there. "Just hold me," I said. I soon calmed down, but what a terrifying night. Never before had a movie affected me so deeply.

After the transplant, and especially after the "ghost" dream, I was far less frightened of death. Now that I had looked death in the face, it was no longer a stranger to be feared. Having been to the brink, I now saw death in a more detached way — as a natural part of life, rather than a terrible misfortune. Death was moving and even profound, but in most circumstances it wasn't inherently tragic.

In my attempt to rejoin the world, I was surprised at how difficult it was to reclaim the level of spirituality I had attained during my illness. I was eager to preserve the lessons I had learned then, including forgiveness, a deeper connection with myself, a sense of composure, and a trust that the universe was unfolding as it should. But my journey back to this world as an earthly presence was extremely difficult. Now that I was healthy and strong, I could almost feel my spirit receding. Although I tried to retain it, some of my spiritual energy was slipping away. I was coming down to earth, my old world, with all its mundane problems.

While I continued to meditate, I now added a brief, daily morning prayer, "Thank you, God, for today," that helped put everything in perspective. Together with the meditation, these five simple words allowed me to move from this physical world, with all of its numbing details and problems, to at least a moment or two of clarity, appreciation, and remembrance. I still repeat this prayer every morning, and at other times during the day, when these words bubble to the surface of my consciousness, I pause to remember where I used to be, and to acknowledge where I am now. And I feel grateful.

Not every aspect of my readjustment was painful, difficult, or frightening. Some changes, especially the physical ones, were thrilling. I remember running to catch a bus; it was almost a block away, and for the first time in ages I didn't stop to think about my condition. I just *ran*. When I was on the bus, and I realized what I had just accomplished, I was elated. I could actually do this!

If I was surprised, other people were shocked. Often they just wanted to touch me, as if to affirm that my recovery was real. Sometimes they wanted to commend me for my "courage," and while I enjoyed the ego-boost and appreciated the compliment, I didn't feel I deserved it. Is there anything courageous or brave about making the only possible choice that will save your life? When you're drowning, you grab any hand that's offered. To me, bravery is a spontaneous decision to save somebody *else's* life when your own is in danger. And yet I was proud of the transplant, and of my persistence in getting through it.

Some people seemed to expect that I would be hooked up to machines, or using a wheelchair; they couldn't quite believe I was walking around, or that I didn't look like a frail old lady. I could understand how they felt, because I couldn't quite believe it myself.

Overall, my physical recovery was more powerful, more successful, and more free of complications than I ever thought possible. After my illness, I would have been more than satisfied to return to anything near the condition I was in before I developed PPH. But I went far beyond that; after the transplant I was healthier than I had ever been in my life. Because of my old heart condition, I had never felt entirely free to run, to play, or even to dance without limits. But now I noticed that without any fanfare, these lifelong restraints had quietly disappeared.

It was remarkable: two years after the transplant I found myself, at the age of fifty, with more stamina and energy than I'd had at twenty-five. I felt like the man in the old joke who asks, "Doctor, after this operation, will I be able to play the violin?"

"Absolutely," says the doctor. "I guarantee it."

"That's wonderful," the man replies, "because I never could before."

What's more, I was granted the unique privilege of bearing witness to my own progress in a vivid "before" and "after" comparison. Back in 1979, several years before I developed PPH, I had performed the lead dance role in a local production of *Oklahoma!* Thirteen years later, and well after my transplant, the music director and the choreographer from that production teamed up again to put on the same play. When I dropped by the audition to see my old friends, they suggested I try out for my old part. Strictly as a lark, I got up on stage. I was flattered when they offered me the role, but the idea of my playing Laurie in the famous dream sequence seemed a little ridiculous. Laurie is very young, and I thought I had been too old to play her *last* time! But my friends kept pushing me, and the more I thought about it the more the prospect excited me. Finally I said yes — not only because it appealed to my ego, but also because this was a thrilling and unusual opportunity. I haven't checked the *Guinness Book of World Records*, but I'm willing to bet that very few dancers have ever performed the same role with two different hearts!

After the transplant, I simply had more energy — a *lot* more. I now felt a new and unfamiliar restlessness, which still hasn't gone away. I was always moving around, looking for somewhere to go or something to do in a ceaseless attempt to stay busy.

Sometimes Amara had to remind me to get enough rest. For all my love of parties, I used to go to bed fairly early. But after the transplant I seemed to be turning into a night person.

So maybe it's not surprising that I found myself spending more time with younger people and less time with friends my own age. I still had my social group from before the transplant, but increasingly, I was attracted to people who were younger than I was. I also noticed that the men who were flirting with me were considerably younger than they used to be. Perhaps it was my heart, and this new presence that seemed to come with it. Or perhaps I was unknowingly projecting my increased libido — a change that has affected almost every transplant recipient I've known, especially if they received the heart of a younger donor. Once, in the supermarket, I saw a tabloid whose headline read *Woman Gets New Heart, Goes Sex Crazy*. It was ridiculous, but it did contain a grain of truth.

As I slowly grew accustomed to this new me, I felt funny being out in the world as a fifty-year-old woman who carried within her the heart and lungs of an eighteen-year-old boy. How weird and amazing it was to have something so close to me, so known to me — and at the same time so mysterious. How was this heart affecting me? Who was this new being I had become? And what did it mean to be the recipient of a miracle that, well within my lifetime, had been the stuff of science-fiction novels?

On the most basic level, it meant I had to be extremely careful. Because of the antirejection drugs I was taking every day, I always had to be vigilant about potential threats to my immune system. When I returned home from New Haven, I lived in terror of my first sneeze. Ever since childhood I had been susceptible to colds, which generally developed into flu, bronchitis, or other complications. Now that my immune system was suppressed, even a couple of sniffles could expand into a life-threatening illness.

So I took precautions. I stayed away from people who were sick with infectious diseases. I washed my hands more often than before. I was especially careful around animals, and also around children, who often carry germs. A friend of mine, a heart recipient who had been a real risk-taker in her former life, returned home from the hospital and learned that some of the students in her children's class had come down with the chicken pox. Although her own children were healthy, at her doctor's suggestion she moved them temporarily to her mother's house, just in case. The doctors and nurses at Yale had made it very clear to all of us: we could never be too careful.

It was about a year after the transplant before I caught my first cold, and when it finally came I was petrified. I'm going to die from this, I thought. Sure, it's only a cold now, but a cold can turn into the flu or bronchitis, and from there I would experience a steep and precipitous downhill slide.

But nothing like that happened. I had a runny nose and a sore throat, and two days later it was over. Instead of feeling worse, as I used to, I quickly got better — just like normal people do. It could have been due to the antibiotics I was taking every day, but the other people in my support group took these same medications, and some of them were often getting sick. I still catch the occasional cold, but ever since the transplant — knock on wood — I seem to have developed a new and welcome resilience. These days, a cold is just a cold.

On one of my periodic checkups back in New Haven, I told Dr. Baldwin that I was no longer plagued by many colds, or by my once-frequent episodes of bronchitis. "That makes sense," he said. "During your transplant, we cut out part of your bronchial tubes and gave you part of his."

So that explained it. Or did it? In any case, it was weird to hear that I had been given even more of my donor's body than I had known about. Dr. Baldwin would have laughed at my own hypothesis, which was that perhaps my donor's heart and lungs, and his vitality, were helping me to heal so quickly. If, by some miracle, I ever made contact with his family, I hoped to learn whether my donor had been as resilient and as resistant to infection as I now appeared to be.

It took years before I realized all the ways that my health had improved. Before the transplant, I had suffered from severe migraine headaches with the classic symptoms: memory loss, visual auras, and one-sided numbness — almost like a miniature stroke. Over the years I had tried a variety of medications to relieve these headaches, but none of them had done the job. The migraines used to occur about once a month, and when I was younger, I was always afraid of getting one before or during a performance. It finally happened during a production of *A Midsummer Night's Dream,* where I forgot a few of my lines and had to bluff my way through by making up some new ones on the spot.

After the transplant I never had another migraine. This may have been due to the cyclosporine, or perhaps even my age, because migraines often fade away as you get older. Not every change I experienced was necessarily a direct result of the transplant, but because organ transplants are relatively new, there are still many unanswered questions.

I had suffered from low blood sugar all my life, but after the transplant this problem also disappeared. So, too, did my life-long aversion to humidity. Until the transplant, I couldn't stand to be in a hot, humid environment; I would feel weak and dehydrated, as if all the energy were draining out of me. But today I can dance for hours in places where, in my previous life, I could hardly have breathed without air conditioning. Before the transplant I never used to sweat, which may explain why I had so much trouble with humidity; my body failed to release enough moisture. After the transplant, I began to sweat profusely during hot weather or strenuous exercise. It sounds funny, but because I wasn't used to sweating, or to body odors brought on by exercise, I had to find a new and more powerful deodorant.

One of the nicest changes of all was that I no longer felt cold all the time. I was finally getting enough oxygen. During my first winter back home, I actually enjoyed going for walks as long as I was dressed for the weather. Every October, as the leaves started falling from the trees, it was reassuring to know that I would no longer be spending the long months between November and April preoccupied with hating winter, or wondering when spring would finally deign to make an appearance. And while I still fantasized about some future move to a warmer climate, for now, at least, I could survive the New England weather, and even enjoy it.

Several other changes were the result of the medications I was taking. The steroid prednisone is known to cause increased facial hair, and my eyelashes grew so long that when I put on my glasses there seemed to be little room left for my eyes. With my nose hair and ear hair growing in thickly, I wondered whether I might at some point have trouble with my breathing or hearing. Fortunately, my facial hair stopped growing after a while, but the hair on my head came in fuller than ever, and it grew so fast in other places that I now needed electrolysis on a regular basis.

So not every change I experienced was directly related to this other presence within me. Some of them, I'm sure, had other explanations — such as almost dying, or being reborn. Other changes came from the medications I was taking, and still others might have happened anyway as I got older. But I find it hard to believe that these other explanations can account for all the things that now seemed different in my life.

The more aware I became of my changing preferences and personality, the more I wondered about my donor. Had he been strong and resilient? Was he, by any chance, hyperactive? If so, that might explain my new and almost frenetic energy. What was his medical history? Would I ever learn *anything* about him? And how, if at all, did my actual donor correspond with the Tim of my dreams?

Eleven

Change of Heart

THE EXHILARATION I felt during and after my first dream about Tim carried over into several other dreams. In a curious reversal of conventional religious symbolism, I dreamed first about rebirth and resurrection, and only later about death and crucifixion — including one nightmare where I actually pulled nails out of my hand. But before these destructive images began, I went through a year of grace when I focused mostly on the thrill of survival. It was as if the exalted magic of my miraculous operation was working as an anesthetic, keeping the negative images away.

In one of my first dreams after the transplant, a man I cannot see is sitting behind me. He talks with me and admires me, but he doesn't allow me to turn around and look at him. When I finally do turn around, I notice that his hands and face are scarred. But I don't find him ugly or repulsive at all. As I caress his hands and face, I find him beautiful.

The man with the scars was a teacher, although I wasn't yet ready to learn his lesson. For the first year or so after the transplant, I couldn't allow myself to face the emotional pain of the operation or its nightmarish aspects. Later, I came to realize that the only way I could come to terms with the transplant was to focus not only on the miracle, but on the darkness as well, including my long illness, the trauma of the operation, and my changing identity. In other words, I had to turn around and accept my scars.

Eventually I did, with my dreams leading the way. As soon as that first year had passed, my dreams became noticeably darker and more violent, with frequent images of bloodshed, war, and other horrors. In one dream I was hiding under the bed in a house that had just been invaded by enemy forces. Right above me was a horrible screeching noise, which sounded very familiar. When I awoke, my first association was the surgical saw that had sliced through my skin at the beginning of the transplant. Although I had been in a far-off world during the operation, maybe on some distant level I had heard that noise. In the dream it was terrifying.

In another nightmare, I was trapped in a cavelike pit in the ground, part of a large group of naked, thin bodies. All of us were huddled together, awaiting the end of the world in this ghastly place that was reminiscent of Auschwitz. Soon all the air would be gone; it was just a matter of time. The image was so awful that I still shiver when I think of it.

When these nightmares persisted, I knew I couldn't ignore them. These images were coming from some deep place within me, a place I obviously needed to explore. In my former life, Rick Pisani had once suggested that if I ever wanted to work on my dreams in depth, the man to see was Robert Bosnak, a Jungian analyst who taught a seminar on dreams at the Jung Institute in Boston. But when I contacted the institute to register for Bosnak's class, it was already full. I then called Bosnak directly to ask if he could take me on as a private client, but he said he was completely booked and had no openings.

"Could you recommend somebody else?" I asked. "I had a

heart-lung transplant, and I want to work on the dreams I've been having ever since."

A pause. "You had a transplant?"

"Yes, last year."

"Really? I might have an hour on Tuesday afternoon."

I liked him immediately. Robbie, as I now think of him, struck me as vital and alive, and his dark eyes seemed to glow with empathy and intelligence. He was also a careful and attentive listener, especially when I talked about the transplant. During our initial meetings, whenever I mentioned the transplant or its effect on me, he seemed almost transfixed. And he was so well informed on the subject that I wondered: Was he, too, a recipient? Was his wife or someone close to him on a waiting list?

When I finally asked him about it, he told me that for the past couple of years he had been writing a novel about a man who undergoes a heart transplant. To learn more about the subject, he had recently picked up Mary Gohlke's book about her transplant, and he happened to be reading her story when I called. Synchronicity strikes again!

It was amazing enough that Robbie was reading Mary Gohlke's book, but the story he was *writing* was even more remarkable. His novel, I learned later, was about a psychiatrist and his girlfriend who are both victims of a violent attack. The girlfriend is killed, and the psychiatrist is so badly wounded he requires a new heart — which she provides. When he finally recovers, the psychiatrist realizes that he is feeling and reacting to events differently than he used to, as though his girlfriend was still influencing him. He gradually comes to know her from the inside, as it were, through the surprising responses of his new heart, which used to be hers.

For a long time, Robbie didn't mention the powerful similarities between his novel and my own story. As a professional, he didn't want his own imaginings to color his client's thoughts and interpretations. During our initial sessions, he said only that he was putting his book aside because he preferred to concentrate on my experiences than on his own imaginative speculations.

That gave me an idea. Because I was keeping a dream journal, and because Robbie had recently published a book called *Dreaming with an AIDS Patient*,* I boldly asked if he might be interested in teaming up with me on a book about the dreams and psychological responses of heart transplants. Robbie liked the idea, and although we both recognized that a literary partnership would infringe on the traditional boundaries between therapist and client, the subject seemed so exciting that we agreed to try it. We would continue my "dreamwork," as Robbie called it, on a different track, although it was clear that the research and the dreamwork would sometimes intersect.

To broaden our scope, we also planned to study the dreams and emotional responses of other heart transplant recipients. At the time, I was still driving to New Haven every month to attend meetings of the support group I had started with Gail Eddy. But by now the group's focus had shifted: there was less emotional sharing and more exchanging of information. I wanted to recruit a handful of participants who might prefer a smaller, more intense research group where, under Robbie's guidance, we could explore our complicated feelings and share our dreams.

For a year and a half, Robbie and I met once a month with six heart transplant recipients in New Haven. This was the group I had yearned for ever since the operation, a small, intense community where we could speak openly and candidly with each other about the full range of our feelings, joys, and fears. Some

---

* This book has been reprinted in paperback as *Christopher's Dreams*.

of our discussions were full of sadness or anger, but always, the sense of being understood made it worthwhile. We could tell each other anything — including private feelings and speculations that we wouldn't share with outsiders, who would probably think we were crazy. We talked of transplant life — and death.

In different ways, we all believed that receiving a new heart had affected and even changed our identities. Robbie and I were both struck by the fact that the participants in our group often referred to themselves not as "recipients," but as "transplants" — as in "I am a transplant." One man, who had previously undergone open heart surgery, with its baffling array of bypasses that resembled the spaghetti of the Los Angeles highway system, insisted that a transplant was a qualitatively different experience. The rest of us agreed: one procedure allows the patient to achieve his normal life span, while the other implies that this life span has been extended beyond its normal limits. This may explain the strong identification with the operation itself. A transplant is not only a transformation of your identity; for a while it *becomes* your identity.

Not only was I finding a voice for my innermost feelings, but so were the others. We were being helped in this process by a man who himself had not experienced a transplant, but who was readily accepted into our exclusive little club as if he had. All of us felt we had finally been granted permission to express the terror, the guilt, and the devastation caused by this horrendous ripping apart and being put back together. We were a little society of Humpty Dumpties.

Being able to talk about these painful subjects was a tremendous relief, because almost everybody in our lives, from doctors and nurses to relatives and friends, felt that we should be eternally grateful for this miraculous gift. And while we *were* grateful, it was terribly frustrating that nobody who hadn't gone through a heart transplant seemed to understand how the depths of our gratitude met the dark places in our soul during the long, complicated healing process. If we were to survive, we needed to understand *all* the forces battling each other within us, from the euphoric ecstasy to the plunging terrors.

All of us, we discovered, were resentful when well-meaning friends and relatives insisted that we ought to be happy and grateful for our transplants, as if it were that simple. What did *they* know about the pains and problems we had gone through? Of *course* we were grateful. We all knew people who had died before or after a transplant, or whose recoveries were terribly difficult.

But we didn't always *feel* grateful. Much of the time we felt rotten, or confused, or frightened. Sometimes our gratitude was obscured by the terrible fears and traumas we went through after the transplant, which most of us could discuss only in the privacy and intimacy of this little community. As one participant put it, "I'm so damn sick of people telling me I'm lucky to be alive. I feel terrible! I'm still getting over a period when I would have had to rally just to die."

Another member described herself as "the nice little woman at dinner parties who understands what kind of conversation people want to hear. They don't want to know I'm sick. No matter what I'm feeling, I have to keep the conversation light. You can't imagine how many times I've been on the phone talking nicey-nicey, and then I've hung up and felt like killing myself. All I can think of is that I must have had a hell of a good time in my previous life."

And a third: "Sometimes I wonder if I did the right thing by having the transplant. Last night I saw a TV show about animals who were injured, who were kept alive until they could be slaughtered. Sometimes I feel like that. If I have to spend the rest of my life preoccupied with staying alive, what's the point of living?"

Another theme in our conversation was that all of us had some sense after the transplant that we were not alone. And each of us had at some point spontaneously experienced our new heart as an "other" with whom some form of communication was taking place. In a couple of cases, this sense of being with another person was so strong that the recipients became obsessed with learning the donor's identity. When this proved to be impossible, the recipients became frustrated and angry at the transplant authorities.

With other participants, the feelings of another presence within were more diffuse and took the form of people talking to their new hearts directly, and sometimes even aloud, during moments of crisis. One man, for example, would tell his heart prior to a biopsy, "Remember, now, we have to cooperate. If we fight, it will kill both of us." To a greater or lesser extent, each of us saw the new heart within us as representing a separate being. Sometimes a discussion between two members would suddenly take on a different tone, as if their two hearts were interrupting to carry on their own discussion.

Only one participant, a social worker named Mary, claimed that she never experienced her new heart as "other." But within the confines of our tight circle, Mary spoke movingly about how, when she experienced an episode of rejection shortly after her transplant, an image came to her of two spirits who were fighting inside her body. "One of them was me," she said, "and the other, I guess, was the donor, who didn't want me to have this heart. I know my new heart came from a woman, and this struggle between us felt like a catfight."

During this period, Mary dreamed that her dead grandmother appeared to her with a message: "Just give something away and you'll be all right." Mary took this to mean that she had to stop fighting for control of her heart and start dealing with the fact that it wasn't entirely hers. When she did, her health improved.

Even so, Mary told us, she occasionally spoke directly to her heart in blunt and unequivocal terms: "You belong to me now. You were somebody else's heart, but now you're mine." These were provocative words from a woman who insisted that nothing unusual or mysterious was going on within her.

Thomas, who was in his forties, took on a completely new personality after the transplant. Before the operation, from all accounts, he had been shy and introverted. But when he joined our original support group a few months after his transplant, Thomas, who now wore a baseball cap all the time, had turned into a big, exuberant, talkative child, like a nine-year-old boy in a man's body. His wife would bring him to the meetings, and he was completely dependent on her. Fortunately, Thomas's extreme regression was only temporary, and during the course of our meetings he regained his old maturity as if he were growing up right in front of us.

Thomas had been told that his new heart came from a teenage boy who was killed in New York. From the start he assumed his donor had been black, although this was never confirmed. Thomas had come from a prejudiced background, but after the transplant he became far more comfortable with black people. He even became enamored with one of the hospital nurses, who looked a little like Tina Turner — the first time he had ever been attracted to a black woman. He started identifying with blacks in general — not only African Americans, but Africans as well. Thomas was surprised to find himself affected by a news report about civil strife in Ethiopia. "I read that blacks on both sides are shooting each other," he said. "They're even shooting at the people who are bringing in relief supplies to save other black people who are dying of starvation. Before the transplant I wouldn't have paid any attention to a story like this. But now it enrages me."*

Thomas told us that his vocabulary had changed since the transplant, and that he had started swearing in front of his wife, which embarrassed him terribly. His language reminded him of his army days, when his speech had been full of vulgarities. Given these changes, I was surprised that he didn't seem very interested in trying to learn more about his donor's identity.

"Sometimes I think about this person whose heart I have," he said, "but I have to put it out of my mind because it scares me. I sometimes picture the doctors standing over his body, waiting for that moment to take his heart, and a couple of hours later putting it in me.

"I won't go so far as to say that two people exist in me, but I have been changed. It might be different if I had received a new kidney, but the heart has spiritual, psychological, and emotional attachments. I believe my donor's spirit is still around, and in that sense he's still alive."

Mario, an energetic, blunt-spoken former shipbuilder in his early fifties, had received the heart of a man half his age. Before

* This statement brings to mind the remarkable story of a Grand Dragon in the Ku Klux Klan who, after learning that his new kidney came from the body of a black donor, responded by joining the NAACP. See Owen S. Surman, "Psychiatric Aspects of Organ Transplantation," *American Journal of Psychiatry*, vol. 146, no. 8 (August 1989), pp. 972–982; p. 977.

the transplant, Mario had suffered from painful episodes of angina, but despite all the agony he had endured, and although he didn't think of himself as especially religious, Mario wouldn't agree to the transplant until his parish priest assured him that it didn't violate Church doctrine. When organ transplants were first performed, Mario had been opposed to them: "Fixing things is fine. But replacing things? I didn't think that was right. And yet I wanted to stay alive."

After the transplant, Mario and his wife noticed a number of changes in his habits. He had never liked bananas before; now he did. He had rarely bothered with dessert; he now loved sweets. And while he had previously been fastidiously neat, after the transplant he was far more relaxed. Mario's wife found these changes perfectly understandable: "Of course he's different. There are genes and energy in him from somebody else's body. Those things affect you."

In at least one respect, Mario's experience was the exact opposite of mine: although he knew very little about his donor, he was convinced he had received the heart of a couch potato, and that this new heart was slowing him down. "I have the feeling my donor's heart isn't strong enough to take care of me. I'm sure he was a professor or somebody who sat around a lot and probably didn't care for my kind of life. I've always been on the go."

An enthusiastic dancer, Mario reproached his donor for ruining his dance rhythms, and he said he was teaching his new heart how to dance. "I lost my ability to dance," he told us. "It's never fully come back to me. I've even yelled out in public a couple of times that I didn't know how to dance — that *he* didn't know how."

Mario also believed that his new heart had undermined his former skill at horseshoes. He loved the game, and until the transplant he had been very good at it. But he was now dismayed to find his tosses were going sideways instead of end-over-end, and that some of his throws were falling short. Here too he would openly rebuke his heart for screwing up. "You dumb bastard," he'd say. "You can't even reach the pit."

About a year after his transplant, Mario had an experience that really shook him up. He and his wife were visiting relatives in the Boston area, and on Easter Sunday they walked into a little church where, to his astonishment, Mario felt completely at home. Even the priest looked familiar, and Mario instinctively knew his way around. He led his wife upstairs to a certain pew, as if he had been there often.

"Have we ever been to this church?" he asked her.

"Never," she replied.

"Well, I have," he said.

"I never knew what part of Boston my guy was from," Mario told us, "but that morning I had no doubt that this was his church." Mario found the experience so unsettling that he returned to the little church three more times until he felt comfortable. "I believe there's another spirit in me," he concluded, "and that we finally bonded together and somehow made a life for both of us."

Mario was especially grateful to Robbie for helping him deal with a disturbing image that kept haunting him. Ever since the transplant, Mario sometimes saw the image of a face suspended just below the ceiling. After one of our meetings, Robbie met privately with Mario and asked him to bring the face into view. When it appeared, Robbie guided Mario in bringing the image down, closer and closer to his own face, until the two faces seemed to merge. After this, the mysterious face made no further appearances, and Mario felt that he had fully integrated the new organ into his body. It reminded me of my own experience after the inhaling dream, except that in Mario's case the merging had been brought about deliberately.

Dorothy, a short, friendly-looking woman with dark hair, was the only other member of our group to have had a heart-lung transplant. But although this made for a bond between us, our post-transplant experiences were totally different. While my physical recovery had been close to perfect, Dorothy had experienced serious problems with her new lungs right from the start. But throughout her long ordeal, she was positive, courageous, and optimistic. In Dorothy's situation I might have felt jealous of me, but although this was the kind of group where jealousy and other awkward feelings could be expressed safely, Dorothy seemed to feel only love and support, not only for me, but for the others as well.

Because the problems were confined to her lungs, Dorothy was able to experience her new heart as benign. In one particularly vivid dream, she traveled through her own blood vessels, a voyage she described to us in glowing terms, like a *National Geographic* special. "This was my way of getting away from all those needles and tubes in the hospital," she said. "Nobody else could go there. When I reached my heart, it was red and pulsating, soft and beautiful. It's a great feeling when you're in there and you know it's you, and that your heart is really working."

Dorothy had been told that her donor was a man, and when things went wrong she thought of her new lungs as still belonging to him. She felt betrayed by her donor because his gift had failed to improve her health. "I probably should feel grateful," she said, "but when something goes wrong, I want to say to him, 'I thought we had a deal! If your lungs had been better, I wouldn't be going through this. You were supposed to be so great you could give somebody else a life. But look what you're doing to me!'"

Dorothy's troubles mounted until the only thing that could have saved her was a second transplant. But in a decision we could all understand, she didn't want to take her struggle any further. "I think it's actually worse the second time. People think it should be easier, but it's not. This time I'm totally aware of everything I'll be going through.

"A few days ago," she told us, "they didn't think I would make it. Everything was so peaceful and I was very accepting. Then I woke up, connected to all these machines. I wanted to say, 'Wait, leave me alone! I've been preparing for this, and I'm not afraid.'"

Dorothy soon became too sick to attend our meetings, and when she died, it was terribly sad for all of us. Shortly after her death, our research group ran out of steam. There were other problems, too, but the death of a member we all loved was a huge loss that we never got over.

Lorna was in her early twenties, with blond, curly hair. She was the youngest member of our group, and, at four years and counting, the longest survivor. She was also the only recipient whose donor had been older than she was, which may be why Lorna felt more mature after her transplant. But she was understandably bitter that her youth had been stolen away. "When my friends and I turned twenty-one," she told us, "they were all having parties. I just wanted a heart. After the transplant, my friends dropped away. People my age couldn't relate to me anymore, and they didn't like the way I looked." Lorna had gained a lot of weight from the medications, and her face was quite swollen.

She was one of the first women anywhere to have a baby after a heart transplant. The doctors had warned against it, but Lorna and her husband had decided to take that chance. Lorna knew her donor had been a woman, and she wanted desperately to tell her donor's parents that she was taking good care of their daughter's heart. But the transplant authorities wouldn't allow her to contact them directly, which was terribly frustrating for her.

Lorna had heard from the social worker that the donor's family had donated the heart after learning that the potential recipient was a young mother with a baby. "I believe my donor was, too," Lorna said. "I wrote to the family, and although they'll never know my name or where I live, I let them know that my little girl was now four, and that I recently had another baby. I thought it might bring them some happiness to know I was making good use of my new heart."

Of all the heart recipients I've known, Lorna had the most terrifying experiences. After her transplant, she was confronted with ghostly images that were so spooky and unearthly that they kept her awake at night. She desperately needed psychological help, but the hospital had no program to provide it. This was another major concern in our group: while society had invested millions of dollars in the advanced training and technology that are necessary to perform these medical miracles, when it came to the emotional and psychological ramifications of this dramatic, life-saving surgery, recipients were essentially on their own.

One afternoon, Robbie asked Lorna about the ghostly figures she had been seeing:

"It started out with images in my mind."

"What kind of images?"

"Images of a woman and a man carrying a young child. Then I see this woman lying in bed on the respirator, with her parents around her. I just know they're her parents. That image comes during the day.

"Then it started happening at night when I couldn't sleep. I haven't slept much since the beginning of all this. When everyone is asleep and I turn off the TV, I look in the doorway and see the image of a white shadow. It's the image of a woman. I believe it's the donor."

"What does the shadow look like?"

"It comes toward me, never touching the ground. It has no feet and no face, just a cloudy image that doesn't frighten me. It comes very close to me, and then it disappears."

"Does it have an intention?"

"I can't figure it out. But sometimes there are two more images. They're dark, and they scare me. They have knives or a gun or an ax or something, and they want to hurt me. They keep coming closer and closer. They come in the doorway and stand over my bed, as though they're trying to tell me that I shouldn't be there, or that I shouldn't have lived. The friendly white cloud is trying to tell me something, and the dark images are trying to scare me.

"Finally I just said, 'Leave me alone!' I said this a few times, and now it's back to just seeing the white image again."

"Can you say more about the identity of these black beings?"

"They're hooded, and they don't really have a face. No definition of arms. I always get a chill when I see them. They never touch the ground; they're always in the air. They come from my daughter's bedroom across the hall, or from the hallway. They come quickly to the door, and then very slowly from the doorway to the bed."

"Is there any other sensation besides seeing? Do you hear anything? Smell anything? Feel anything?"

"No, I just have a sense that they want to harm me, or warn me about something. They stand above the light. If I turn on the light they'd go away. But I freeze. I can't move. I want to yell, but I can't make any sound. Sometimes I turn to my husband and ask, 'Did you see that?'"

"And has he ever seen them?"

"No, he never has." She sounded disappointed.

"And is their presence as tangibly real as this chair, or is it another kind of reality?"

"Another kind. I can almost see through them."

"So they're phantoms?"

"Yes, like a ghost."

At the very least, Lorna's harrowing experience reflected her ambivalent feelings about the transplant. It had given her life, and she was truly grateful for the new heart. At the same time, it appeared that the demons wanted her to die, which may reflect the part of Lorna that felt unworthy of this gift.

Of all the participants in our group, I was closest to Joseph, a handsome musician in his early forties with curly red hair and a beard. After years of living with debilitating coronary disease, he finally received a new heart, and joined our original support group a few weeks later. Although Joseph wasn't much of a talker, his warmth and humor made him an instant favorite. His wife came with him to our meetings, and we all became fond of this warm and loving couple.

Or so we thought. Within a few months, however, Joseph was coming to meetings alone. His wife left him six months after the operation, and he was miserable. Although none of us had seen it coming, what happened to Joseph wasn't unusual. As

I had already learned the hard way, a long, serious illness can put an enormous strain on even a good relationship. Some recipients go through years of marital problems, and both parties agree — sometimes explicitly, but often without saying so directly — to keep the marriage going at least until after the transplant. In other cases, the recipient undergoes a significant personality change after the operation, which can mean that the entire relationship has to be reconstructed — no simple matter. As I became increasingly aware of the painful details of other people's breakups, there were times when I was almost relieved that my relationship with Alan had ended when it did. The task of readjusting to the world after a heart transplant is stressful and complicated enough without the additional burden of trying to cope with the effects of a traumatic breakup.

Joseph, too, had received the heart of a much younger man. He played baseball, and after the transplant he injured his arm more than once because he now threw with such strength that his body couldn't handle it. Not surprisingly, Joseph's dreams, like some of mine, expressed the theme of a youthful heart trapped in an old body that couldn't keep up. In one dream, he was a young player, riding the bus to a game with his teammates. But when the bus arrived and everybody ran to the field, Joseph was left behind; his body was so old and crippled that he had to crawl off the bus.

Later, in a striking series of three dreams, Joseph was able to visualize the successful integration of his new heart. In the first dream he was in a wheelchair, unable to walk. In the second, he was behind the wheelchair, pushing it along the road. In the third and final dream, he folded up the wheelchair and put it away. A dream sequence rarely comes out so clearly, but what a wonderful feeling when it does.

Because Joseph's transplant was in late October, he was in the ICU over Halloween. That night, Joseph dreamed that he begged to be let out of the hospital in order to go trick or treating. It was, perhaps, an odd request for a man in his forties, but this was a dream, where anything is possible. The hospital authorities allowed him to go as long as he didn't stay out too late.

The next morning, the nurses were astonished at Joseph's output of urine, and one of them jokingly asked if he had been drinking beer all night. "I must have peed about a gallon," he said. "It was as if this kid went out drinking, and as a result I was peeing all morning."

As soon as he awoke that morning, Joseph wrote, "He wants to come out. I could feel his force, holding my fists, running his course." This was a common feeling among us — a claustrophobic sense of being held down while some living force within us was desperately trying to escape. I had this feeling in the hospital, when I felt my heart wanting to leave the confinement of this strange new body.

About a year after Joseph joined the group, and after we had been friends for a while, our relationship became romantic. Because of what we had both been through, this was far from a typical courtship. On our first date, for example, we met for cyclosporine-and-milk cocktails. Apparently this was how heart-transplant recipients went out for a drink.

Although Joseph lived in Vermont, he often drove to Boston to see me. On one of those trips, we went out to dinner with his sister and her husband. Joseph's brother-in-law was driving, and Joseph and I were sitting together in the back. Our driver had a bad cold, and at one point he sneezed several times in a row. When we heard those sneezes, Joseph and I didn't need further instructions. Like most transplant recipients, we each carried a surgical mask, just in case. And now, without a word, we instinctively reached for our masks and strapped them on. We must have been quite a sight, sitting there silently in the darkened backseat, holding hands and wearing those little white masks. When Joseph's sister turned around to ask him a question, she could barely suppress a scream.

It was comforting and even romantic to be with a man who had exactly the same health concerns I did, which led to at least one other amusing moment when we had breakfast together at a little neighborhood diner. Like me, Joseph took more than a dozen pills each morning, and even more at night. After placing our orders, we began lining up our pills, just as we did every morning. By now this routine was so much a part of our lives that we continued talking while our fingers did the counting and sorting. When the pills were in place, we casually took our plastic plungers, which looked like little syringes, and started injecting cyclosporine into our juice.*

When I finally looked up, our waitress was staring at us in open-mouthed dismay. Just as I was realizing what this scene must have looked like, she said, with real worry in her voice, "Excuse me — you guys aren't planning to shoot up, are you?"

We began explaining that we weren't drug dealers or even drug *users*, but that we were taking all these pills because both of us blah blah blah. . . . But I had the impression that our words rang false, and understandably so. Trying to convince a nervous waitress that one of her healthy-looking customers had undergone a heart transplant was already asking a lot. But *two* customers?

While I normally took my medicine at home, every now and then I had no choice but to swallow my various pills on a plane

---

* This experience is now outdated, as cyclosporine is available in pills.

or in a hotel dining room, which always made me feel as if I were on display. To be able to go through this routine with another person made an enormous difference, and to go through it with someone I loved — well, that was marvelous. Joseph and I really saw each other as soul mates. Or perhaps, in our case, heart and soul mates.

With all the medications we were taking, not to mention our respective transplants, we often joked about the "chemistry" that existed between us. We had each received the heart of a much younger person, and in our more intimate moments there was an amazing vitality between us, as if there were four souls in the room instead of two.

Joseph and I had a deep spiritual connection that was sometimes reflected in our dreams. One night I dreamed about a little boy who was drowning and sinking peacefully into the sea without a struggle. Each breath became more shallow, until finally the boy let go. The people on the shore became frantic. They wanted to save the boy, but they couldn't find him in the water. Meanwhile, Joseph stood next to me on the dock, quietly confident. The two of us seemed to share and know something the others didn't, which allowed us to remain calm and peaceful.

Then Joseph extended his foot in a magical, elongated way, and made contact with the boy beneath the water. He tapped his foot lightly on the boy's chest where his heart had been beating. Then everybody tried to save the boy. They grabbed him from the sea and began to resuscitate him. Now the hard part began. Out of that peaceful letting-go, the drowning boy was thrust back into life, gasping for air and finally beginning to breathe again.

There were two important themes in this dream. First, I loved Joseph because he was the only one who understood, as I did, what the boy was facing. Only someone who had gone through a near-death experience can fully appreciate how difficult and painful it is to be yanked back to life when a peaceful death is imminent.

But the dream had another meaning, too. When I explored it with Robbie, he helped me understand that despite my powerful drive to survive after the transplant, some part of me had still not returned to life — until now. There is a place in our souls that can be touched only by love — the love of somebody who truly understands us. Joseph touched that place in me and helped me be fully alive, just as he had touched the boy's heart in my dream and brought him back to life.

We started having similar dreams — and even crossed dreams. I used to have recurring dreams about a dog who spoke to me, and although Joseph and I sometimes discussed our dreams, I had never mentioned this one. One morning Joseph told me he'd just had a dream in which I had a dog named Freddie who suddenly began talking to him. Wow! Now I knew the name of the talking dog in *my* dreams. This experience marked a new level of intimacy for me, and it made me love Joseph even more.

But things change. I was alone in my kitchen one morning when a cool breeze blew in through the open window, scattering napkins and papers from the table. When I stood up to close the window, a little crystal heart that Joseph had given me fell to the floor and shattered. My heart was broken! I tried to glue it back together, but it wouldn't hold. On the spot, I sat down and wrote a poem about the shattered heart. While it wasn't Shakespeare, it was the first time in my life I had written a poem.

I wondered, of course, whether the breaking of this glass heart might be a portent of what lay ahead for us. I was afraid it was. Our attachment was so close and powerful that Robbie, who knew Joseph from our research group and liked him a lot, had given me a prescient warning: "I'm truly happy for both of you," he said. "But it may be that this relationship turns out to be so intense that one of you feels compelled to run."

Joseph ran. In the summer of 1990, when I turned fifty, Amara and Danny made a party for me. I invited fifty-one guests — one for each year, plus one more for good luck. I invited Joseph, too, although he was beginning to pull away from me. We still lived in different towns, and he had recently been spending time with another woman. Joseph didn't say so directly, but I had the feeling our relationship was ending.

After the party, Joseph and I spoke in broad, general terms about how amazing it would be if two heart recipients ever decided to get married. But our discussion remained theoretical.

Several weeks later, I heard from mutual friends that Joseph's new companion had moved in with him. I was crushed — not only because it was over between us, but also because Joseph hadn't told me himself. Although I was enormously disappointed, I didn't dwell on it. I survived a transplant, I told myself. I'll survive this, too. My heart can take it.

Months later, when we finally talked it over, Joseph acknowledged that our relationship really had been too intense for him. But although we didn't end up together, I'll always feel a special attachment to him. We loved each other, and had a unique bond that neither of us is likely to experience again. Joseph remains deep in my heart, and I expect he always will. From time to time I still listen to a tape he made for me, where he sings a song he composed shortly after his transplant. The song is called "Change of Heart."

Twelve

Heart Throbs

SOMETIMES a situation has to become worse before it gets better. When I first started working with Robbie on my dreams, I was often buffeted by strong feelings and unexpected impulses. During this period I made a couple of decisions that were reckless and out of character, but which seemed to fit into a larger picture of my relationship with the elusive Tim that was slowly coming into focus. Eventually my life would stabilize, but the path to my new identity wasn't always smooth.

I had just begun working with Robbie when I became enchanted by a dazzling new man. Kirk was tall and lean with light brown hair, and when we ran into each other in a local park, I could almost see the sparks between us. He looked to be at least ten years younger than I, but if that didn't bother him, it certainly didn't bother me. After a long conversation that neither of us wanted to end, he asked if I would join him for lunch.

A few days later Kirk invited me to his house. As I came in, I noticed a prominent display of trophies.

"What are these for?" I asked, expecting to hear about his prowess in tennis or his passion for golf.

"I won them racing motorcycles," he said. "That's one of my hobbies."

Okay, I thought. Younger man, light hair, motorcycles —
what exactly is going on here?

Somehow we were talking about ice skating. I have always
loved to skate, and I mentioned to Kirk that I was looking forward to winter so I could get back on the ice.

"You don't have to wait," he said. "Let me show you something."

He walked over to the closet and pulled out two sets of
Rollerblades. Handing me the smaller pair, he urged me to try
them on. I had never Rollerbladed in my life, but the skates fit
and Kirk's energy was seductive. Moments later I was sailing
down the hill outside his house. I was exhilarated, but slightly
self-conscious. Wasn't this a sport for younger people?

Kirk didn't think so. But in his eagerness to get me up and
rolling, he had neglected to teach me how to stop. Moments after it began, my maiden voyage came to an ungainly and bumpy
end as I coasted right into a parked car at the bottom of the hill.
Although I was bruised, I was having too much fun to care about
the pain.

A couple of days later I ran into one of my neighbors on the
street. "You know," she said, "I thought I saw Amara Rollerblad-
ing the other day. Then I wondered if it might have been you,
Claire. But that couldn't be, not after the transplant, right? It
doesn't make sense."

No, I thought, it really doesn't. But that was precisely what
had made the experience so enjoyable. Kirk didn't make much
sense either — not for a woman my age, with my interests. And
yet I couldn't stay away from him.

Kirk was divorced, owned his business, and was obviously
doing well. He was playful, glamorous, and constantly on the
move. A devout hedonist, he had made his house into a real
bachelor pad, complete with Jacuzzi, hot tub, and even a

waterbed. This guy's idea of a casual supper consisted of sizzling steaks and chilled martinis by the fireplace. He reminded me of the type of man who used to read *Playboy,* and who saw the magazine as a practical guide to the good life.

He was, in short, totally unlike any man I had ever been attracted to. And yet I was intensely attracted to him from the moment we met, before I knew anything about him. I felt that we shared the same energy in our hearts. But as much as I enjoyed being with him, I didn't feel I knew him. One thing I could never understand was that although Kirk had been adopted, he had never been interested in searching for, or even learning about, his birth parents. Maybe I was projecting my own growing curiosity about my donor, but I was baffled by his apparent indifference to his origins.

Near the end of our time together, I had a bizarre and disturbing psychic experience. It began with a dream: the doorbell rang at Kirk's house, and a young, attractive woman named Suzanne came in and asked for Kirk. He greeted her warmly and took her upstairs to show her the bedroom.

The next morning, while I was writing down the dream, I asked Kirk if he knew anyone named Suzanne.

"No," he replied. "Why do you ask?"

"Oh, just a dream," I said, without revealing any further details.

Just then the doorbell rang. Kirk went to answer it, and I heard him say, "Hi, Suzanne." This was too weird! Kirk introduced us, and although he had met this woman only recently, I could feel the erotic charge between them. When Kirk took her upstairs to show her the rest of the house, I started shaking. This was so frightening I had to leave. Before they came back down, I put on my boots and ran out of the house. I was sure that my days with Kirk were numbered, and they were.

Our liaison was electric, dramatic, and brief. Like a bright flame of passion, the romance fizzled out soon after it began. From the start, my attraction to Kirk seemed to emanate from some new and unfamiliar place within me. During our few weeks together, I was happy to join him in his continual, almost compulsive craving for action and excitement. And while I had been active ever since the transplant, with Kirk the pace of my heart seemed to be turned up a notch. It was now expressing a new energy all its own, with an intensity and a drive I could barely keep up with.

Naturally, I talked with Robbie about how my attraction to Kirk seemed to be related to the transplant. Kirk, after all, looked a lot like the dream image of my donor. Robbie pointed out that when I met Kirk I had just started working on my dreams, so it was likely that my image of Tim had shifted to the front of my consciousness. As soon as I found a man who seemed to embody that image, I was hooked — even before I learned about the motorcycles. As I suspected, my intense and inexplicable attraction to Kirk was really a projection of my imaginings about Tim — whom I idealized. Kirk, you might say, was my dream lover. When he turned out to be less than ideal, I was distraught.

But even after Kirk was gone, that youthful energy remained alive within me, searching for another outlet. I continued to experience an intense craving for action and speed that seemed connected, somehow, to my new organs. And why not? My lungs regulated my breathing and my heart controlled my pace, so wasn't it possible that their presence within me might have a profound effect on my rhythm?

A few weeks later, when I was still unable to contain my restlessness, I impulsively flew off to France. But instead of going to France like a middle-class, middle-aged lady, I was more like a college kid on a summer break. I spent hours sitting on the floors of dusty train stations, waiting for trains among knapsack-bearing students on their way to youth hostels. Clothes were strewn about, sleeping bags and backpacks were everywhere. I had been to Europe before, but never like this, not even when I was younger. At the age of fifty I was dashing around France at a frantic pace — and for no apparent reason.

It should have been fun, but mostly I felt confused. What are you doing? I kept asking myself. Why are you traveling like this if you're not enjoying it?

The best answer I could give was that my heart seemed to be leading me here. It sounds a little nutty, but that's how it felt. My body was exhausted, but this powerful boy's heart kept pushing a tired, middle-aged woman. My heart seemed to be in command, while the rest of me — the older me — was barely keeping pace with it.

Parts of that week were pure misery. Nobody helped me with my lousy French, or with the heavy bags I lugged up long flights of stairs to the train station. When I finally made it to the top, nobody could tell me where to buy my ticket. There were lines everywhere, and the entire population of France seemed to be choking on cigarettes, stinking up the air I needed to breathe.

As I breathlessly dragged my luggage from one track to the next, I was frequently lost and continually confused. What train am I looking for? Where will I find it? Am I on the right track? Long after my body was exhausted, my heart kept pushing me on.

When I finally stumbled into the right train, I fell into an animated conversation with my seat mate, a warm and gregarious dark-haired man in his twenties from Brooklyn. As we rode together through the long, dark night, he was so attentive that I unburdened myself and babbled on about the miserable time I was having. Ever since landing in Paris a few days earlier, I had felt invisible to the French, partly because I didn't speak their language. Now, for the first time in days, I felt *seen* — even in this dark train.

When he saw I was crying, my companion started stroking my arm. "Would you like me to hold you?" he asked. I could feel my youthful heart leaping toward him. Although I was old enough to be his mother, this unexpected invitation conjured up a romantic reverie of a woman alone on an overnight train in a foreign land, who is suddenly swept up in the arms of a handsome young stranger.

Who's in charge here? I wondered. Is it me, or is it my heart? And who am I, exactly? Daring traveler or prudent parent?

This time my head prevailed over my heart. While I had some tempting fantasies of where this encounter might be headed, I didn't act on them. This is your life, I told myself, not an Erica Jong novel.

The following night, safely ensconced in my hotel, I lay in bed and wondered what on earth was going on with me. What was I doing here, thousands of miles from home, from the hospital, from Amara? What if something happened? Were there any transplant doctors in France? And why had I come over here in the first place, to this utterly foreign place, with foreign currency and a foreign language, where I didn't even know how to use the telephone? Ever since the transplant, I had been feeling foreign even to myself. Why did I increase the burden by adding even more foreignness to my life, and especially by traveling alone?

The older, rational me was asking these questions, but that wasn't the same person who had purchased the airline ticket to Paris. It wasn't my old self who had dragged me here, but the youthful energy of my now twenty-year-old heart and lungs. In

France, more than ever before, I felt as if I were two people who were sharing the same body.

I was reminded of the wonderful movie *All of Me,* where the soul of an older woman (Lily Tomlin) transmigrates into the body of a younger man (Steve Martin). But because his body now contains two different personalities — male on one side, female on the other — this poor, confused man is forced to re-learn his identity. In one extremely clever scene, the two sides of him try to cross the sidewalk together, each in its own way, which leads to a preposterous tug-of-war. Although the division within me was not nearly so obvious, when I saw the film again after the transplant, it really touched me — especially the parts about getting used to another presence within you. It was just as funny the second time, but a lot more believable.

Not surprisingly, this struggle within me was also reflected in my dreams, which were increasingly concerned with Tim. Among the first topics I had discussed with Robbie were the dreams about babies, including the ones I'd had a month or so before the transplant. Why babies? Because after my donor died — and even before, for that matter — I had symbolically brought him back to life. As Robbie put it, "A new self was born in your dream world."

As time passed, Tim began appearing in other guises — not only as a baby or a young man, but also as a boy. In one dream, I'm on a passenger ship, where I'm involved with a family with two young boys. The younger boy and I have a special rapport, and he seems to have a crush on me. He draws a red rose and offers it to me as a gift. Then it becomes known on the ship that the boy has died. Although nobody on board wants to talk about it, I know that his death had something to do with me.

"What do you feel now?" Robbie asked as we worked on the dream.

"A lot of sadness. I'm all choked up. I can feel it in my stomach, my throat. I don't know whether it's longing, regret, or gratitude."

"And it has something to do with the little boy giving you his rose?"

"Yes, he's giving me something very precious of himself." Then I recalled a time many years ago, when I drew a rose on a piece of paper and gave it to my husband, together with a loving inscription. It was the same rose I had seen in the dream.

"What were you thinking, or writing, when you gave the picture to your husband?" Robbie asked.

"With love from my heart, with all my heart — something like that."

"So in a way the little boy is giving you his heart?"

"Yes." There was no question about it. The boy with the rose was another manifestation of Tim, whose death most certainly had something to do with me.

In another image from this period, it was Tim's *life* — his energy and vigor, that was affecting me. One spring morning, the day before I was due at Yale for my annual stress test, I was stretched out on my long, brown velvet couch, eyes closed, doing my daily meditation. I had just reached a deep state of contemplation when Tim appeared to me — as if in a dream. He was healthy and young, and he wore jogging shorts, a tee-shirt, and sneakers. He was on a treadmill, running in place, just as I would be doing tomorrow. He was sweating profusely, as if he were training for some kind of Olympic event. He was on top of the world and raring to go. His intensity and drive were pumping through the room.

The next day, during my stress test, I could feel his boundless energy within me. I was walking faster and faster up a simulated hill, and the technicians were amazed at my endurance. So was

I. This fifty-year-old woman was being propelled forward in this youthful dash, like the older Margot Fonteyn dancing with the twenty-year-old Nureyev. It was as if this boy and I were now a single being, whose heart and lungs were so strong we could go on indefinitely, as if I had a new, permanent, and internal dance partner.

Eventually my legs gave out. My muscles and my old body just couldn't keep pace with the younger parts of me. What was left of Tim was valiantly pumping my blood through a body that couldn't match his vigor. For a brief moment I felt his future that was never to be, and his youthful spirit trapped in a body that couldn't contain it.

Although Tim could have stayed on the treadmill forever, the technicians had to stop the test. Exhausted, I was led into another room to watch the sonar video of my heart. The dye injected into my blood during the stress test made my circulation visible, and I could actually see how I was Tim and Tim was me.

Here again I was experiencing the transplant from the perspective of my donor. As my journey progressed, I was increasingly aware of the other side of this equation. How shocking it must have been for Tim's heart and lungs — and whatever parts of Tim's spirit that might have come along with them — to wake up in the body of a middle-aged woman. Was I crazy, or were my dreams and my changes suggesting that the human heart was more than a mechanical pump?

Thirteen

Mystery Dinner

IT STARTED OUT like any other weekend. In August 1990, on a humid Friday night, I went to a mystery theater dinner with my friend Anne and my nephew Stuart. At nine o'clock, as dessert was being served, I began lining up my pills and injecting my nightly dose of cyclosporine into a small container of orange juice. People often turn away when they see me taking my medicine in public, but my table mates that night were friendly and open, and were watching me with real interest. Somebody asked if I had just robbed a pharmacy, and when I explained why I was taking all these pills, I was flooded with questions about the transplant.

Later on, one of the unattached men at our table came over to continue the conversation. Fred, a handsome fellow who was visiting from Florida, introduced himself as a "rainbow maker." As we talked, I wondered whether Fred was genuinely interested in the transplant, or was using it as a way to flirt with me. Or perhaps both.

"Do you know who your donor was?" he asked.

"Not really. Just that he was an eighteen-year-old boy from Maine who was killed in a motorcycle crash."

"Nothing else?"

I explained that the hospital officials would not release any other information, and that strictly speaking, I already knew more than I was supposed to.

When Fred persisted, and when he told me he was especially interested in dreams, I took a chance and described the dream where I had kissed and then inhaled the young man named Tim L., whom I thought of as my donor. Although Gail had implied that this wasn't the right name, the dream was so powerful that I still believed it.

Fred was fascinated by this dream, and he pressed me for additional details. He told me he had psychic abilities, and I nodded politely. This was beginning to feel like a come-on. But there was something about this man that I liked, and when he asked for my phone number, I gave it to him.

He called the next morning, and was eager to get together. When I told him (truthfully) that I was busy all day, he said, "There's something I want to tell you. I dreamed last night that I saw your donor's obituary in the middle of the page of a Maine newspaper."

Well, *that* got my attention. Although I still wasn't sure about Fred, who was I, of all people, to be dismissing other people's dreams? It sounded like a long shot, but why not check it out?

"Here's what we could do," I suggested. "I'll call the Boston Public Library to see if they have any newspapers from Maine. If I don't call you back, let's meet there at two o'clock."

As I was looking up the number of the library, I wondered why it had never even occurred to me to search for my donor's obituary on my own. After all, I knew the date of death, I knew the young man's age, and I thought I knew his name. And yet the idea hadn't entered my mind.

"Maine is a big place," the librarian told me, "and we carry only one newspaper from the entire state. Frankly, it sounds like a wild goose chase. But if you'd like to come in and have a look, just ask for the Microtext Department."

I arrived a little early. Fred was already there, scrolling through the newspaper for the week of my transplant. I stood behind him and peered over his shoulder as the pages slid by.

Oh my God! There, in the middle of the page, was the item we were searching for!

I felt a sudden weakness in my knees.

"That's it," I said, collapsing into a chair. "It's him."

I was sure of it. The date corresponded with my transplant, and the details matched what little I already knew.

He was eighteen. The cause of death was a motorcycle accident. And his name was Timothy Lasalle.*

I felt weak all over. So the first Tim dream was true after all!

But now what? The obituary, which I photocopied, mentioned five sisters and two brothers. Here was the family of my heart on a piece of paper. What do I do now?

Until this moment I hadn't been 100 percent certain that the transplant had even happened. The whole process had been so otherworldly that it was almost easier to view it as a miracle. The fact that I wasn't allowed to know my donor's name and address only added to the feeling that this had been a mythical event. Until now, most of my information about the donor had come from images and dreams that were difficult to decipher and impossible to confirm.

---

* At the family's request, I have changed their names and the name of their town to protect their privacy. Tim's last name, however, did start with an "L." The first sentence of the obituary read as follows: "MILFORD — Timothy Lasalle, 18, of 29 Chestnut Street, died Friday at a Bangor hospital from injuries received in a motorcycle accident in Milford."

Suddenly I knew that the donor was real, and that he had a family. Now there was proof: a name, an address, a town.

Fred and I went to a nearby coffee shop, where Fred was full of questions. What was I going to do now? Was I going to contact the family?

I told him that I didn't know, but that this was something I definitely wanted to think about. I thought I would write them a letter, but I didn't want to act hastily. As we left the coffee shop and went our separate ways, I said goodbye to Fred and thanked him warmly for helping me. I had met this man only yesterday and would probably never see him again, but today he had potentially changed my life. What mysterious force had brought this "rainbow maker" into my life? How had he come to have that dream? Was it just a coincidence that the library carried this one Maine newspaper, or had Fred been dropped on my path in order to connect me to Tim's family?

I was tempted to call Gail immediately, but I decided to wait a few days. I was going to New Haven anyway, and I wanted to tell her in person. Besides, I wasn't sure that Gail could add much to what I had just learned.

But I did tell Robbie, who was very excited about the obituary. In a way, he was even more affected than I was by this tangible evidence that Tim had really existed. Although Robbie was empathetic and open-minded, until he actually saw the obituary he had insisted on seeing Tim only as "Tim" — that is, as a dream presence, designated by quotation marks, who might or might not have had a connection with my donor. To Robbie, "Tim" was a psychological event, and what mattered was my experience of him.

But now Robbie was forced to consider what had long seemed clear to me — not only that there was a "real" Tim, but that some aspects of him might exist within me. As Robbie wrote:

I feel a change of viewpoint taking place. My vehement attachment to the psychological point of view about "Tim" is loosening up as Claire comes closer to her desire to meet with Tim's family. I am beginning to believe that some of Tim's essence has transmigrated to Claire. As a professional therapist, I know that vigor and resilience are part of character, temperament, and identity. If the transplant has somehow passed on elements of his temperament, personality, and identity, then psychological residues of the actual Tim L. (not just the image of "Tim") may now inhabit Claire.

I can feel the quotation marks dropping away as I leave the safe confines of psychoanalysis and move into the tricky realm of belief.

In New Haven, I had dinner with Gail.

"Remember when I called and described the dream where my donor appeared?"

"Of course I remember."

"Well, I know now that I had the right name."

She looked at me. "What makes you so sure?"

"I found his obituary in a newspaper, and it was the name I gave you from the dream."

She sighed. "Claire, when you called that day I wasn't sure what to tell you. Your call really spooked me. But I couldn't confirm the donor's name because it was just a dream."

I told her about Fred's dream, and how he had led me to Tim's obituary. As I described it, I wondered if she believed me. At this point I wasn't altogether certain that *I* believed me.

"Let me ask you something that might explain some of this," I said. "Do you think it's possible that Tim's name was spoken by one of the doctors during the surgery, and that it somehow reached me in my unconscious state?"

"I was wondering the same thing," said Gail. "It's the only way I could explain it. But the doctors never mention the donor's name; they're not even aware of it. Besides, your transplant was my first time in surgery with Dr. Baldwin, and I remember it clearly. It was so quiet in there you could hear a pin drop. That's how Dr. Baldwin works: not a word is spoken."*

We moved on to other topics, but as our dinner ended, Gail repeated her earlier warning that it might not be a good idea for me to contact the family.

"I don't know what I'll do," I told her. "Right now I'm just sitting with this information. I haven't contacted them yet, but it's something I definitely want to think about."

One of the few people I told about the obituary was John, a hospital chaplain in Boston who counseled families of accident victims and was often asked to provide information and advice about organ donation. John and I were friendly, and from time to time we would lecture together. He would explain the process from the perspective of the donor's family, while I would describe what it was like to be on the receiving end of an organ transplant.

If and when I contacted Tim's family, I thought of John as a potential intermediary. If the family was willing to meet me, I wanted to drive to Maine with Robbie and John — or at least one of them. Despite the pull I was feeling to go there, I didn't want to make the trip alone. I was too frightened — of the un-

* This wasn't only Gail's impression. "Unlike many surgeons, Baldwin doesn't speak much while operating," observes Sherwin Nuland in a detailed account of a heart transplant at Yale–New Haven Hospital. "The scene reminded me of nothing so much as one of those old Hollywood movies in which the two skilled safe-crackers are working with exquisite care and no overt signs of hurry but always against the ticking of the clock." Sherwin B. Nuland, "Transplanting a Heart," *The New Yorker,* February 19, 1990, pp. 82–94, p. 90.

known, of how I would be received, and of my emotional reaction. And theirs.

John was eager to be involved. "I could contact a friend from that area," he said. "He'll find out what he can, and perhaps he can even be in touch with the family on your behalf."

When a week passed with no word, I called John again.

"Were you able to talk to your friend?" I asked.

"Yes," he replied. "He wasn't able to contact the family directly, but from what he picked up, I think we should abort the trip."

Abort? A strange choice of language for a minister, I thought.

"What do you mean?" I asked.

"This is hard for me to tell you, but apparently nobody was surprised when Timothy died. He was known for driving fast. I'm not sure about this, but I get the impression there were other problems, too. Maybe drugs or alcohol. This kid lived on the edge, and my guess is that he had a lot of problems."

"Oh my God." It was terribly hard for me to hear that the young man I had been imagining and seeing in my dreams might have been very different from the person whose heart and lungs had become part of me.

"I'm sorry to be telling you this, Claire, but that's what I was able to come up with."

I was devastated. Numb. My hero had just been torn down. Alcohol and drugs? Wait a minute — didn't they screen organ donors for those problems?

Gail's earlier warning was ringing in my ears: *Don't open this can of worms.* Why hadn't I listened to her? One thought led to another, and soon I was wondering whether Gail knew more about this family than she was letting on.

I called Robbie to tell him the latest. "I don't think we should proceed any further," I said. "This is too painful for me."

"Why? Because the real Tim may not have been wonderful? Maybe he drank. Maybe he had other problems. Everybody has a dark side."

But I wasn't ready to hear this. "I think we should abandon our search," I said.

"It's up to you," he said.

During our next session, Robbie and I talked again about how I had been carrying around an idealized image of Tim. Although he respected my decision to pull back, Robbie urged me to keep an open mind. "People are complicated," he reminded me. "The real Tim was probably a complex person with a mix of good and bad qualities. Do you really want to abandon your search because he might have been different from the fantasy figure in your dreams?"

Robbie was in a delicate position. Ever since I had found the obituary, he was excited about visiting the family. Assuming they agreed to see us, this would be a marvelous opportunity to learn who Tim L. really was, and whether he corresponded at all to the "Tim" of my imagination. But while Robbie didn't want me to give up too hastily, he also made no attempt to pressure me.

For a week or two after my conversation with the chaplain, I was terribly sad. I immersed myself in this new information and allowed it to wash over me.

And of course I had a dream: I am in an elevator with other people, facing a dark man whose back is against the wall. He is wearing a dark blue sweater. I place both my hands on his chest and say, "Timmy, you are my brother."

I couldn't have scripted it better. After my initial fear about the real Tim's possibly sinister side, the dream Tim had darkened and turned blue. The tall, golden-haired figure I had

dreamed about earlier was transformed into a solid, less idealized, and more substantial character. The image was less romantic now, and more realistic. I had accepted this man as my
brother. And if that were true, then Tim's family was also my
family. Despite my fears, I seemed to be taking another big step
in their direction.

The blue sweater in the dream had an additional significance:
during the winter months, Robbie invariably wore a blue
sweater. This merging of Robbie and Tim wasn't surprising:
during my analytic work with Robbie, I often projected aspects
of Tim's invisible presence onto him. The transference that I experienced and examined with Robbie made it easier to explore
my feelings toward Tim, and even to form a relationship with
him. In a sense, Robbie, too, was my brother, who was joining
me in my search for Tim. Ever since the obituary, my bond with
Robbie had grown stronger as we circled around Tim in ever
smaller loops.

The blue sweater dream carried a strong message of acceptance, and a couple of days later I overcame my earlier reserva-
tions. Robbie was right. Even if the chaplain's information
about Tim was true, did that mean I shouldn't contact the family? Perhaps what still existed of Tim was his purer essence. If he
had been tormented in life, he was free now to fly — and he
seemed to be doing that through me. As I turned these thoughts
over in my mind, I was gradually coming to terms with Tim —
whoever he turned out to be.

I called Gail with a question: "If a donor were addicted to
drugs," I asked, "or had been drinking a lot, how would that affect his heart?"

"I'm not qualified to give you a medical answer," she said, "but
I can assure you that before a donor is accepted, the medical

team runs a lot of tests. Nobody wants to go to the enormous trouble and expense of transplanting an organ that may not be healthy. I'm not exactly sure what you're getting at here, but your donor's liver was also donated, so it must have been healthy. As far as I know, there was no hint of any problems."

Gail's answer helped, and so did Robbie's comments. But what really made the difference was my allowing the issue to percolate for a couple of weeks. When I emerged from this process, Tim was more my hero than ever. I was convinced that some part of him was living within me, and was somehow leading me to his family. Sooner or later I expected to contact them, and when the time was right I would know it.

Life goes on. When Amara finished high school and my child support ended, I gave up my Brookline apartment and moved back to Hull, a few miles south of Boston. The house sits on a cliff overlooking the ocean; when I'm there, it feels like I'm literally living on the edge. Before I was sick, Amara and I used to spend weekends and summers here. During my illness I had stayed in Brookline, but I never stopped thinking about that peaceful and calming place on the ocean, with its magnificent views of the water.

I moved back to Hull on May 1, 1991. That very night, I dreamed about Tim. He was wearing a black cape, and was about to ascend to a high place that looked like the horizon.

"Where are you going?" I asked him.

"To die," he replied. "I'm going to the other side."

"What's it like over there?"

"Oh, I come right back."

He was pretty sure of himself, and had apparently done this before. Going back and forth seemed to be a routine adventure for him. As in the ghost dream, walls and boundaries that were normally solid had become permeable.

So Tim was following me — following me to Hull, and also leading me to his family. The very day I moved here, to a house with a sweeping view of the horizon, Tim had appeared in a dream about the horizon. As soon as I awoke from this dream, I knew it was time to contact the family. Almost nine months had passed since I had found the obituary, but I had yet to act on it.

But now the barriers were down. If Tim could move back and forth between worlds, so could I.

On my second night in Hull, I dreamed about a young man who has been seriously impaired since birth. He wants to be with me forever. We go to his home, where his family is, and we tell them we'll always be together.

This dream, right on the heels of the other one, reinforced my decision to contact the family. An impaired young man — who, in another realm, might be reduced to his heart and lungs, wanted to be with me forever. This was reminiscent of my very first dream about Tim, where I inhaled him into me, knowing that we would be together forever. In this latest dream, we had gone home together to visit his family. If that wasn't a signal, nothing was.

As I saw it, Tim had done everything but send me directions to his parents' house.

So I wrote them a letter:

Dear Mrs. and Mrs. Lasalle:

With the passing of another year, I write once again to thank you for the gift you have given me. No words can properly express my gratitude. This has been a very productive year for me: working on a book about heart transplants, the performance of a new work I have choreographed, watching my daughter enjoy her first year of college, and just thoroughly enjoying the simple, ordinary things of every day, something I no longer take for granted. I have also begun a support group for people who are recipients or candidates for transplants.

The authorities did not give me your name or address. That knowledge came to me in another way, and I have taken the liberty of writing to you personally.

If you do not wish to respond, I understand. If, however, you, as I, would like to communicate, you can reach me at _____, or by phone at _____.

Gratefully yours,
Claire Sylvia

A few days later I drove to New Haven for the monthly meeting of our research group. Because our sessions began in the morning and generally lasted most of the day, I used to drive down the previous afternoon and stay over in a hotel. On the morning of our meeting, I was awakened by a phone call from Amara, who was staying with a friend.

"Hi Mom, you had a few calls on the machine yesterday."

"Anything important?" I asked.

"Well, I thought you might want to know that Mr. Lasalle called."

Really? While I had hoped and even expected that Tim's family would respond to my letter, I was so excited by this news that I momentarily forgot where I was, or what I was doing in this hotel room. Then I glanced at the clock and saw that our meeting would soon be starting. I ran to take a shower.

As I was drying my hair, Robbie knocked on the door. He had just driven down from Boston, and he looked exhausted.

"Wonderful news," I told him. "Mr. Lasalle called."

"Really? What did he say?"

"I didn't speak to him. Amara gave me the message."

"Any indication that they want to see you?"

"He didn't say. Amara was at a friend's house, so the number's at home. I'll call tonight when I get back."

Back in Boston, my friend Pam suggested that I return Mr. Lasalle's call from her house so I wouldn't be alone. She settled me on the couch with a glass of wine.

"I'm incredibly nervous," I told her.

"Tell me about it," she said. "Why did you write to the family? What makes you want to visit them?"

It was odd to hear the question put so rationally. Until now I had been operating mostly on instinct and intuition.

"I feel as if somebody else is inside me, and I want to know who it is. I also want to make a connection with Tim's family."

"Why?"

Why indeed? I hadn't really put this into words before, but I found myself telling Pam — and also acknowledging to myself — that ever since we had moved out of my grandparents' apartment when I was young, I had always wanted to be part of a big, warm, loving family. Maybe Tim's family was like that.

"And one member of that family is gone," Pam said.

"Yes, he's gone, and I'm here instead. Or maybe he's here, too, in some way. I have this feeling that Tim has been leading me home, and that my going to see his family might be his way of coming back to them."

Pam smiled. She was asking big questions, but my concerns at that moment were small and practical.

"When they answer the phone," I asked her, "what should I say?"

"'Hello' would be nice."

"No really, what am I supposed to say to them? *Hello Mom and*

Dad? I'm partly your son?" Soon we were giggling like nervous teenagers.

Finally I picked up the phone. As I punched in the numbers, I could hear my heart pounding.

Ring.

How long should I wait? Maybe they won't answer. Or maybe I *hope* they won't.

Ring.

Maybe I shouldn't be doing this. Maybe Gail was right.

Ring.

Every moment was adding new anxieties. What if the chaplain was right? What if Tim was a drug dealer? What if I hung up now?

Ring.

Relief. It seems they're not home.

Ring.

No, wait, be home, *please.* Don't make me go through this again!

Ring.

No answer, no machine. Well good night, Tim's family, wherever you are. I hung up feeling let down, my body sagging.

"Go home and get a good night's sleep," Pam said. "Try again tomorrow, and make sure there's someone with you."

With another friend, I tried again on Sunday morning. Again, no answer. Maybe they were in church.

That afternoon, with the call weighing heavily on my mind, I decided to try again. I was alone, but so what? Enough stalling, I told myself. They've got to be home now. Call them and get it over with.

"Hello?" A soft female voice.

"Hello, this is Claire Sylvia."

"How are you?" Very matter-of-fact, as if I called them all the time.

"Very well, thank you. Thank you so much for calling the other day. It means a lot. I understand that your family not only saved my life, but several others, too."

"We got together and decided that's what he would have wanted." No mention of Tim by name. Was that significant?

"How did you find us?" she asked.

I was hoping she wouldn't ask — not yet, anyway. Acutely conscious of her feelings, I began to tell her about the dream where Tim first appeared to me. I spoke slowly, weighing each word. My heart felt jittery, and I couldn't sit still. As I finished, I realized she had been carrying on another conversation that was unrelated to ours. I ended by telling her how I had found Tim's obituary in the library.

"That's a nice story, dear," she said. Although it was clearly said without malice, I winced when she used the word "story."

"And how are you?" she asked again.

Her absentminded response dropped on me like a heavy stone. I don't know what I expected, but it wasn't this. I pushed ahead anyway.

"Would it be all right if I came to visit?"

"Yes." A woman of few words.

Knowing that Robbie was free on Mondays, I asked, "Would a week from tomorrow be all right? I'd like to come with a friend, since it's a long drive."

"Well, I work that day, but you could come anyway and visit my husband." That was odd. Didn't she want to see me?

"Would a Sunday be better for you?"

"Yes, we could do it on a Sunday, if it's later on in the afternoon."

What's going on here? Why hasn't she shown any emotion?

We agreed I would come on the first Sunday in June.

I was laughing as I hung up the phone — not because the conversation was funny, but because I was anxious, and this conversation was so oddly understated and unemotional. I saw myself as offering to bring this woman news of what had happened to her son, but she showed no affect, no enthusiasm, no excitement. Did she think I was loony? Or was she possibly feeling deep emotions and holding them in check while talking to a total stranger on the telephone?

I called Robbie, who said the date was fine with him. Then I called Mrs. Lasalle again to arrange the time and to get directions. Something had changed: "I thought, after we talked, that I could switch with someone at my job, so you could come earlier." This was a relief, the first indication that our meeting might be important to her. But when she put her husband on the line to give me directions, we were back to the land without feelings. He directed me to a parking lot near their house, and said he'd meet us in a brown car. For all he seemed to care, I might have been delivering a truckload of firewood.

Don't make assumptions, I told myself. A lot of people are wary on the phone. They're probably different in person.

June 2 was a very hot day. Robbie and I didn't talk much during the drive, although Robbie did mention that his daughter, a year younger than Amara, thought our trip was "weird." Perhaps Amara did too, although she hadn't said much about it.

"How do you imagine the parents?" Robbie asked me. I had no answer. My mind was blank, and all my previous images of Tim had disappeared. No more troubled teenager, and no more warm family that would sweep me into its bosom. No more prodigal daughter returning home. No preconceptions, although I was glad I was bringing flowers.

I hoped they were eager to see me. While I wanted to thank Tim's family for giving me life, I had heard that the act of donating organs often helps the mourners in their own healing. I wanted to believe that in my small way, I had provided an opportunity for them as well. Although I couldn't imagine how they felt, I believed I was bringing a part of Tim back to them.

"Will the rest of the family be there?" Robbie asked.

"I have no idea."

Eventually we found our way to the parking lot, which was deserted on a Sunday.

"What do you suppose this place is used for?" I asked Robbie.

"This must be the place where transplant recipients meet with their donor families," he replied. We both laughed, breaking the tension.

As we got out of the car to stretch, a brown Toyota pulled into the lot. My heart jumped.

A woman drove up and looked right past us. Her car had Vermont plates.

Then Robbie spotted him. A large brown station wagon drove slowly into view. Robbie waved, and the driver, a man, waved back. My stomach tightened. It seemed to take him forever to park. Finally he came to a stop beside us.

As we got out of the car to meet him, everything seemed silent and dreamlike. Only the squeak of the car door broke the mood.

He was alone. I thought they were both coming, but maybe she wasn't interested. Or maybe she had to work after all.

Mr. Lasalle was smaller than I expected, and he greeted us

perfunctorily. I was bringing him the heart of his son, and he said "hello." I was expecting a profound moment, and he said, "Follow me to the house."

"That was awfully casual," I said to Robbie when we were back in the car. "But at least he seemed friendly."

"He's probably nervous, too." Robbie said. Good point. I was so wrapped up in this moment that I hadn't stopped to see it from the family's point of view.

The world of Tim's parents consisted of freshly mowed lawns and large clapboard houses. Mr. Lasalle pulled into a driveway. To our left, on the lawn, was a stone statue of the Holy Mother of the Sacred Heart.

My stomach was churning. I needed a bathroom. I was breathing quickly and holding on tightly to the flowers.

As we followed Mr. Lasalle to the screen door, his wife came out with a smile. I liked her instantly. Fragile and solid at once, she looked like an accepting presence. My stomach relaxed a little, but my steps were tentative and ambivalent. She looked like the handshaking type, so I reached out to shake her hand. I was surprised — and immensely pleased — when she hugged me instead.

I turned around to introduce her to Robbie. Their greeting was a little more formal, but I could see in Robbie's eyes that he was taken with her.

As we stepped into the house, I felt myself falling over a cliff. And into a whole new world.

Fourteen

Family
of My Heart

ROBBIE AND I followed Mrs. Lasalle into a large, bright living room, where three young women — Tim's sisters — stood up to greet us. When we all sat down, I found Robbie's eyes just to make sure he was there. I was incredibly nervous.

We discussed the heat and the humidity, and the small talk dragged on. And on. And on. Was there any way to stop it? Tim's heart was sitting on Tim's couch next to Tim's mother, and what were we talking about? The weather! And the highways between Boston and here, and whether it was better to take the toll roads.

Meanwhile, of course, we were all sizing each other up. While I was chatting with his wife, Mr. Lasalle was scrutinizing me. Robbie told me later that the sisters were watching me like hawks.

The absence of real communication became excruciating, and I finally excused myself to use the bathroom. When I returned, iced tea was served, and we settled back into our awkwardness. There was an elephant in the room and nobody wanted to acknowledge it. Would the whole afternoon be like this?

We were joined by a young blond woman with ruddy cheeks and blue eyes. This was Annie, a fourth sister, who was closest in age to Tim. Leaning against the mantel, she looked me in the eye and said, "So tell us what you know. What about the dream you told my mother on the phone? And you're writing a book?"

I wanted to jump up and hug her for being so real. But at first we were all taken aback by her directness. She had sliced right through our small talk. Robbie and I looked at each other and laughed.

Annie blushed and said, "Well, I thought I'd better ask."

I assured Annie that her questions were important to me, and that I loved her for asking them. She blushed even more and gave me a beautiful smile.

I sensed that Robbie was startled by her mention of our project. "How do you know about the book?" I asked.

"You mentioned it in your letter to my parents."

That's right, I had. I knew Robbie so well that I could almost see his analytical suspicions beginning to rise. If they know we're writing a book, he was thinking, was all this going to be theater? Would they now portray Tim as totally sunny and flawless?

A shirtless man entered from the back of the house. John was one of Tim's older brothers. Tim's five sisters and two brothers grew up in this house, just as, a generation earlier, Tim's father grew up here with his eight siblings.

Carla turned to her brother and said, "Claire was just about to tell how she found us."

As I began my story, everyone leaned forward in anticipation. My narrative was interrupted at times by soft exclamations of amazement: "Unbelievable," somebody said when I described the inhaling dream. When I finished, eyes were misted over with silent tears.

"None of the other people who received his organs have been in touch with us," Carla said.

"No," said another voice, "the man with the eyes sent us an Easter card." In addition to his heart and lungs, the family had donated Tim's corneas, kidneys, and liver.

"At first," said Mrs. Lasalle, "I didn't want to do this. I didn't want him all cut up." There was pain in her voice.

"It's a good thing we had two days to decide," added one of the sisters, "or we wouldn't have done it. We needed some time to get used to the idea. In the end, we all decided that my brother would have wanted it this way."

"Would you like to see a picture of Tim?" Mrs. Lasalle asked. It was moving to hear her speak his name in my presence.

"Oh yes," I responded. I was *dying* to.

She went to another room and returned with a framed photograph. Sitting back on the couch, she turned the picture so I could see it. I moved closer.

He wore glasses, although I didn't see him that way in my dream. In this photo he looked about fourteen. He was dressed in formal clothes and was standing beside a priest. But even with the glasses, I could see the sparkle in his eyes.

Mrs. Lasalle started to say something about Tim when she suddenly choked up. Now the tears flowed. When I moved to embrace her, I could feel her thin and solid body grieving in my arms as we cried together. I felt a bond between us, a bond like nothing I had ever known.

"Mrs. Lasalle," I began, but she stopped me and said, "Call me June, dear."

"And your husband is Carl?" I asked, turning to him. Somehow, he seemed less solid than his frail-looking wife. He appeared to be on the verge of saying something, but he couldn't allow himself to do it. There seemed to be something unspoken and unfinished between Carl and Tim. It wasn't expressed, but I felt it in my heart.

"Would you like to see Tim's room?" June asked. This was more than I had hoped for. I got up from the couch, my body moving with a will of its own. I turned to Robbie, who smiled and followed us upstairs.

Tim's room looked like the room of any boy. It was in no way unusual, except that it was Tim's room.

June led us across the stairwell to a guest room. On the shelves of a low, open bookcase were photographs of the children, together with their bronzed baby shoes. She reached down for Tim's picture and handed it to me.

I was looking at a five-year-old, whose darling face smiled up at me. I recognized the spirit in those bright eyes; it had been with me since the transplant. He was such a little boy in my hands, so full of life and of mischief.

But I couldn't quite comprehend this, my holding Tim's picture in my hands and his heart in my chest. I paused to take a breath and Tim's lungs filled with air. Except that they were my lungs now. Mine to breathe with, as I grieved with his mother next to me. Time had stopped for a moment as I stood here with Tim's picture and Tim's mother.

June reached for the photograph, but my hands didn't want to let it go. I clutched the picture to my heart before returning it. Time had started up again.

Back downstairs. In the den off the living room, a framed poem hung on the wall. Tim's older sister wrote it a few days ago, for his three-year memorial service. I realized that while I was rejoicing in the third anniversary of my new life, they were grieving all over again.

As I tried to read the poem, the words floated in front of me through a blur of tears. I was exhausted from all this emotion, and I wondered if my heart could stand it. What if my heart couldn't take it anymore, and I died right now, right here?

No, they can't go through *that* again. I'd better die somewhere else.

. By now the living room was teeming with relatives. Everyone
wanted to meet me and hear my story. Tim's cousin sat next to
me on the couch and asked if she could touch me. I felt little
touches on my hands and arms as if she were making sure I
really existed.

"I was very close to Tim, and I didn't have a chance to say
goodbye," she told me, and we embraced.

Her husband had brought a videotape with some shots of
Tim. They said he was shy in front of a camera, and sure enough
we saw him from the back, repairing a vacuum cleaner but re-
fusing to turn around. His body was thin and wiry, like in my
dream. Then he said, "I fixed it already."

Somebody mentioned that shortly before Tim died, he went
around asking family members if there was anything they
needed done before he left. When I heard the phrase "before he
left," a shiver rippled through my body. Was it possible Tim
knew he was going to die? I thought back to last month's dream,
the one that compelled me to contact the family, where Tim
told me he was going to the other side. "It's easy," he said in the
dream. "I come right back."

Back in the video, Tim was goofing around with his sisters
and making silly faces for the camera. His playfulness reminded
me of the Tim of my dreams.

"He seems very active," Robbie observed. A comment, but
really a question.

June said that Tim had a tremendous amount of energy. The
sisters described how difficult it was to baby-sit him, and how
he tried to run away from them until they tied him to a rope.

"He was restless," somebody added, "holding down three jobs
and all."

I nodded vigorously. This made sense to me. June said that Tim had more energy than any of her other kids.

"That's why he loved motorcycles," one of the sisters said.

I was reminded of my whirlwind trip through France, and how often Tim's heart had worn me down with its constant craving for activity.

"Was he a beer drinker?" I asked.

His sisters nodded. Then his brother said, "He didn't drink that much." End of discussion. I had the feeling that Tim liked beer, but that his brother didn't want us to think so.

When I told them how I wanted a beer soon after the operation, there were smiles all around.

"Did you ever have the urge to drive a sixteen-wheeler?" Josie asked with a grin. "Tim always wanted to drive those big trucks."

"No," I replied. "Well, at least not yet." We all laughed.

"He always wanted to be a truck driver," Carl said.

It was so amazing just to be there that I had to remind myself that I had come with some specific questions. I asked if Tim ever had colds, and whether he recovered quickly.

"He hardly ever got sick," somebody said. "And when he did, he got over it fast."

Not much doubt in *that* answer. Maybe I really did inherit his resilience.

I asked if he liked green peppers.

"Are you kidding? He *loved* them," a sister told me. "He used to fry them up with a whole kielbasa sausage."

I explained that I never liked peppers before the transplant.

"But what he *really* loved was chicken nuggets," said Annie.

"Oh, my God!"

"What is it, Claire?"

"I just remembered something I've never told anyone. After the transplant, when I was finally allowed to drive again, the first place I went to was Kentucky Fried Chicken. I had this craving for chicken nuggets, which I'd never had before."

Everybody laughed. John said that after Tim's accident, they had to remove a container of chicken nuggets from under his jacket. He was carrying them when he died.

The front door opened and Tim's aunt came in. Greeting me, she was close to tears. During the final months of Tim's life, he had spent time at her house after a fight with his father over buying the motorcycle. Tim's aunt didn't stay long. Maybe she couldn't bear the conflicted feelings that my visit had stirred up.

As she was leaving, June's mother arrived — a beautiful woman in her eighties, elegant and tastefully dressed. Everyone mentioned her quick recovery from her recent surgery, and it occurred to me that perhaps Tim's grandmother was one source of his remarkable resilience. And mine, too.

She came right over and hugged me with tears in her eyes. "It's wonderful that you came," she said. "You're part of the family." These were the words I'd been longing to hear, and now I, too, had tears in my eyes. I felt embraced and accepted by this big, warm, loving family, the family I had been longing for, the family Tim had left me.

June handed me a newspaper clipping from 1988. It was an article about my transplant, which included my name and the fact that I lived in Brookline. I was stunned.

"So you knew all along," I blurted out.

"We wanted to be in touch with you, but the hospital people strongly discouraged it." I glanced over at Robbie. He was shaking his head in anger, just as he did when Lorna from our research group described how she had desperately wanted to get in touch with her donor family, and that the hospital officials had refused to help her.

"We were so happy when you wrote to us," June said.

From here the conversation meandered along various lines. Suddenly a question hung in the room:

"What is your religion, Claire?"

I hesitated. What if my being Jewish was a problem for them? How would they react when they learned that Tim's Catholic heart now resided in a Jewish body?

"I'm Jewish."

Silence. Maybe they didn't know any Jews. But when the conversation resumed without a break in the mood, I was relieved.

"Do you want to see Tim's grave?" Josie asked. The idea spooked me; I couldn't imagine what I'd feel like when I got there. But I couldn't turn back now. I had come this far, and now I had to go all the way.

"Yes, I'd like that."

The meeting soon drew to a close. I was hugged and kissed profusely, with standing invitations from all over the state.

We set off for the cemetery. Josie drove, with Carla next to her. Robbie and I were in the back. Along the way, we were shown the neighboring houses of two aunts.

Josie turned around to ask, "Do you want to see where he had his accident?"

Oh God, I thought, do we *have* to? But I said, "Oh, yes." A subtle switch had occurred: until now I had been sharing my experience of Tim, which the family was hungry to hear. Back in the house, an added element of performance came into my story, like the feeling I get when I take the stage and begin dancing. But now the momentum had shifted, and they were sharing their Tim with me. I had become their audience, and I no longer knew what to expect. I wasn't sure I wanted to learn these new steps, or where they might lead.

The sisters pointed out a brown house on the left. "Tim painted it just before the accident," said Carla. "He was proud of his work, and we think he probably turned to admire it just before the other driver pulled into the driveway." Josie stopped the car next to a huge tree.

"This is where it happened," she said. "The woman who was driving the other car had to leave it there. She couldn't get back into it. It stayed there for weeks until they finally towed it away. Just before Tim drove here, he passed our house and Dad yelled out to him to slow down. Dad always wanted him to slow down."

"He flew into that tree headfirst, without a helmet," said Josie. "His brains were all exposed by the time the ambulance came."

I was shocked to hear her describing Tim's death in such graphic detail. I didn't really want to hear it. But Robbie was studying the tree as if he intended to engrave each detail in his memory. I was so glad he had come with me.

As we got back into the car, the air was heavy with emotion. Nobody said a word.

The cemetery was filled with statues — mostly welcoming Christs and consoling Madonnas. I stood in front of Tim's stone, a light-colored polished granite. On the side of the grave, fresh flowers rested in a vase. "Dad brought those," Carla said.

Tim's sisters were down on their knees in prayer. I wanted to put a stone on the marker, the way it's done in Jewish cemeteries, and I asked the sisters if this would be all right.

"Sure," they said. Robbie handed me a pebble, and I performed the little ritual that has been done for centuries. But instead of being overwhelmed with feelings, I was numb.

As I placed the pebble on the headstone, I read the inscription over Tim's name and dates: FOREVER TOGETHER. A chill ran down my spine. I didn't know how that phrase was intended, but for me it had a very special meaning: at the end of the dream where I first met Tim and inhaled him into me, I knew we would be together forever.

I hugged the girls. Now we were all crying.

When we returned to the house, June and Carl invited us for dinner at a nearby restaurant with Josie and Carla. I ordered chicken nuggets in honor of Tim, and the gesture seemed to be appreciated. Now the conversation was light and pleasant, far removed from the purpose of our visit.

"I'm not much of a correspondent," June told me, "so I won't be writing very much. But we want you to know that you're welcome here any time you like."

"We'll write to you, if it's all right," said Carla.

"I'd love that. And you're welcome to visit me any time."

Carl sat back, smiled, and paid the bill.

As Robbie and I walked June and Carla back to their house, June asked if we'd like to come in for a little dessert.

I looked at Robbie. "We'd love to," he said. "But we really should be heading back. It's getting late, and we have a long drive ahead of us." I felt the same way. I didn't want to leave, but I was exhausted.

"Well, okay," she said. "I just made a little cake to go with some coffee."

Robbie and I looked at each other again. "Of course we'll come in," we both told her.

Inside, June disappeared and returned with a huge sheet cake, decorated with a single word in large print: WELCOME.

As the mother of my heart presented the cake to me, her face was beaming.

"Chocolate," she said. "Tim's favorite."

Fifteen

More About Tim

AS ROBBIE AND I began driving back to Boston, I was exhausted, almost too tired to speak. But I was also elated in the afterglow of a truly unforgettable day. I had just learned that many of the dreams, images, and hunches I'd had about my donor matched up closely with what his loved ones knew about him. And in addition to telling me about Tim, they had welcomed me into their family. It was amazing: just this morning, these people had existed for me as one-dimensional strangers, a flat list of names in a newspaper obituary. Now, during the course of a single afternoon, they had sprung to life as spirited, breathing souls. And I was one of them!

As we drove along dark country roads, Robbie and I tried to reconstruct every detail, word, and gesture from our long, emotional, and very satisfying meeting. We had both been taken with Tim's beautiful and stately grandmother, and one of the many highlights of my visit was the way this noble woman had wholeheartedly and tearfully enfolded me into her family. But we had also noticed a certain ambivalence about my arrival, which seemed to break down along gender lines. Tim's mother, his grandmother, his sisters, and his cousin were all happy and excited to meet me, and were clearly open to the possibility that some kind of metaphysical or spiritual connection existed between Tim and me. Tim's father, however, and especially his brother, were more cautious and distant, while two other siblings hadn't shown up at all. And when I said goodbye to Carl, I had the strong sense of unfinished business between father and son. I actually felt it in my heart.

For Robbie, who had observed this odd reunion through more detached and objective eyes, today's encounter had provided an opportunity to test some of his own conjectures about Tim. Above all, Robbie wanted to know whether, as he had predicted from my own behavior, Tim had experienced a constant craving for action during his brief life. From everything his family said, that was indeed the case. Again and again we were told of Tim's tremendous energy and restlessness — ranging from his childhood attempts to run away from his older sisters through his more recent decision to work at several different jobs during his high school years.

Reviewing these stories in the car, we were both reminded of my trip to France, when I had been propelled by a mysterious, manic drive that seemed to emanate from some other source. Now I wondered whether there was any special meaning to the fact that I had ended up in France, of all places. Tim's family was of French-Canadian ancestry. Was that another link, or was I searching too hard?

Some of the things we had learned in Maine were too remarkable to ignore: Tim's love of chicken nuggets, for example, or his fondness for green peppers. And while nobody in Tim's family seemed to think there had been anything unusual about his health, Robbie and I were both struck by Tim's strong resistance to colds and infections. For a healthy person, of course, not getting sick seems so normal that it's not even noticed. To me, however, it feels like a miracle.

The one puzzle that we couldn't solve was how to interpret the negative report about Tim that had come from John, the chaplain. How did John's depiction of a deeply troubled young man fit in with everything we had just learned? It was remotely possible, of course, that Tim's entire family had been acting and putting on a show for us, perhaps without even realizing it. But that scenario seemed unlikely, and from everything we have learned since, the family's description of Tim was accurate. By all accounts, he had been loving, sweet, and helpful. I have to conclude that the chaplain's report was wrong, although why and how that happened remains a mystery.

Over the years, with the help of Tim's parents, his teachers, and his friends, I have been able to fill in a few more details about him. For a long time I was curious about Tim's girlfriend, assuming he had one. I now know that while there was no one girlfriend, Tim did have a big crush on a girl who didn't happen to share his feelings. When she started going out with another boy — a close friend of Tim's, in fact — Tim was distraught.

For years I wondered about this girl. Was it possible that she looked like the type of woman I had suddenly and inexplicably started noticing and staring at after the transplant? Apparently she did. Although I have never met her, I now know that the object of Tim's affections was short and curvy, with curly blond hair. Soon after the transplant, in the dream where I had changed from a woman to a man and then back again, I had seen a girl just like this, who was about to get married. Her image had stayed with me, and I can still picture it today — a face and figure completely different from the taller, darker women I used to find attractive. Could there possibly be a connection between Tim's favorite girl and the woman in my dream?

I also learned that both of Tim's parents, not just his father, had been unhappy about his riding a motorcycle. "I don't want you buying one," June had told him. "You don't need it, and it's too dangerous."

"Ma," he had replied, "if I die on the motorcycle, I'll fly straight to heaven on it."

When I heard that, and especially the word "fly," I thought back to two of my dreams. In the gender-changing dream, Tim had flown right across the highway, into another world. And in the dream that finally led me to contact the family, Tim had been about to fly up over the horizon.

"Where are you going?" I asked him.

"To die," he replied. "I'm going to the other side."

"What's it like over there?"

"Oh, I come right back."

Did the real Tim believe on some level that death wasn't the end? Did he have a death wish? Although I was finally getting some answers, each new answer was leading to more questions.

As June described it later, it had taken some time and a fair amount of consideration before the family agreed to donate Tim's organs. The doctors made their request, and the family discussed it.

"The kids said, 'Ma, what do you want to do?'"

"I said, 'Well, it's up to all of us.'"

Then one of the sisters spoke up. "Listen, if Timmy had a penny in his pocket he'd give it to you, even if it was his last one. That's the kind of person he was."

There was no argument about that. When the family thought about what Tim stood for, their decision was clear. Later, Tim's parents and all of his siblings signed organ donor cards.

During my initial visit to the family, I hadn't realized that Tim was known all over town for his many acts of kindness. Later on, however, I heard stories. The family had a neighbor who was old and infirm. In the winter, in the middle of the night, Tim would take it upon himself to shovel this man's driveway so it would be clean in the morning. At school, when Tim overheard one of his favorite teachers admiring a popular style of sneakers that her students were wearing, he discreetly learned her shoe size and bought her a pair. He brought flowers to another teacher, and earrings for her little girls. He was always giving presents and doing favors. And I heard again how, the week before he died, Tim dropped in on friends, relatives, and teachers to see if they needed anything done. Every time I think about this, it gives me chills. It's as if he knew he was leaving.

I guess it's unavoidable: whenever I learn something new about Tim, I search my memory to see if it corresponds with some change, however minor, in my habits or personality. Was there any link to Tim's generosity? I think so, although it's not especially dramatic. My sister and Ira have both told me that since the transplant I have become more compassionate and thoughtful. I've always enjoyed giving gifts, but I seem to be giving them more often now.

From time to time I still wonder about changes in me that might be related to my new male heart. After the transplant, for example, I lost the desire to cook. I used to have a good touch in the kitchen, but that's no longer true. Is this change related to Tim, or is there some other explanation? I'm also less bothered than I used to be by perceived slights or critical remarks, which strikes me as another move in the general direction of masculinity.

Before the transplant, I had a flair for putting clothes together and coming up with interesting combinations. After the transplant, I didn't know how to dress, almost as if my feminine touch had disappeared. My color preference has also changed: I used to be drawn toward hot colors — red, pink, and gold. I had never liked blue or green and had rarely worn them, but ever since the transplant I've been attracted to these cooler colors, especially deep forest green. I didn't attach any great meaning to this change until somebody pointed out that green is the universal symbol for new life. But it's also true that most men stay away from hot colors, as I now do.

Again and again, people who knew Tim talked about his enormous drive to keep moving. Apparently it started early. At the age of two, he disappeared one morning when his father refused to take him in the car. One minute he was standing on the porch in his diaper; the next minute he was gone. When June couldn't find him anywhere, she frantically called the police station. Fortunately, two girls in the neighborhood had found a little boy toddling down the road.

Later, Tim would channel his love of motion into driving. Even before he had his license, he used to drive a neighbor's car for her. "Don't worry," she told him. "I'll pay the ticket if you get caught." Before Tim bought his motorcycle, he bought a truck and spent his limited free time fixing it up. His friends remember that he loved working on it, and that he was always thinking about the next vehicle he could buy.

He was continually on the go. He hated sitting around, and he didn't like television or going to the movies. He worked relentlessly — mornings, afternoons, nights, weekends, and holidays — doing construction, painting houses, washing dishes, shoveling snow. All over town the verdict was unanimous. "He worked all the time." "He loved to work." "An extremely hard worker." "A workaholic." "Crazy hours." The owner of a food market where Tim was employed recalled that he used to stop by even when he wasn't on duty, almost as if he enjoyed just being *around* work.

Not surprisingly, Tim's many jobs didn't leave much time for school. He skipped a lot of classes, and although he was close with several of his teachers, school was a burden for him. He was good in math, but he seemed to have had a learning disability that made reading difficult. "It's hard to fit into a traditional high school when you can't read and people don't understand that," said one of his teachers. "He was smart and highly motivated. He had another kind of intelligence, and a lot of common sense."

Was Tim dyslexic? If so, that might help explain one of the more subtle changes I noticed after the transplant. I used to be a terrific speller, but in recent years, for no apparent reason, I have been reversing letters. I also take down directions incorrectly, and I mix up the digits in phone numbers. All of this, of course, might be a sign of aging. But while these errors don't occur often, before the transplant they didn't happen at all.

Have I made Tim sound like a saint? He wasn't, of course. Like many teenagers, he sometimes got into mischief. In the eighth grade, he and his friends were suspended for drinking. Once, covered with mud, he jumped into a teacher's swimming pool. He also had a temper, and although he was close with his siblings, he often sparred with them. There were fistfights, too — including some with his father. "He wasn't a discipline problem," a teacher recalled, "but if he felt something wasn't fair, he'd get into an argument."

"He did have a quick temper," said one of his employers. "But after the explosion he'd be very upset with himself. He'd say things and regret them, and he'd end up feeling twice as bad as the person he was angry with."

Despite his temper, people who knew Tim said he was more mature than his peers. He got along better with adults than with people his own age, and one of Tim's teachers still has the receipt for the flowers she bought for his funeral. She can't explain why she kept it, but she can't throw it away, either.

While I was completing this book, a reporter asked Tim's parents about the day in 1991 when I first went to see them. "It made me feel my son came back to me," said Carl. And June concurred. "He might be gone, but in a way he's still around."

"Do you believe," the reporter asked, "that in some way Claire picked up part of Tim's spirit?"

June: "Yes, I believe it. When she told us about the foods, it was a shock. My daughter said, 'Ma, I can't believe it. That's the same stuff Timmy liked.'"

Carl: "His spirit is still there in those parts she received."

A few months after I met Tim's family, a producer from the *Phil Donahue Show* called to ask whether I would come to New York to talk about my post-transplant experience. I've always enjoyed the limelight, and I immediately said yes.

Three of Tim's sisters said they'd be happy to go on with me. When the producer insisted there was room for only two family members, the sisters wouldn't budge. "Either all three of us go on," they said, "or do the show without us." The producer backed down and invited all three — Annie, Josie, and Carla.

There were other guests as well, including Robbie and two members of our New Haven research group. For the sake of balance, the producer also invited a heart transplant surgeon who was suitably skeptical of any experience that couldn't be explained by medical science.

As it turned out, the surgeon wasn't needed. The studio audience provided all the skepticism and hostility a producer could have asked for — and then some. Even the host was sur-prised by their strident negativity.

Early in the program, Tim's sisters described my visit to their family. Annie said she was skeptical before I arrived, because my story sounded like something out of the movies. But when I walked into the living room, she said, "It was like meeting my brother all over again, seeing him alive. Claire was loving like Tim was. There was so much feeling that it was absolutely ex-hausting."

"When we met Claire," said Carla, "we all probed her and asked her questions. It was like she knew Timmy. A lot of things she said were true. How would she know these things? Every-thing she was saying was right. It was just like *him,* like she was part of him."

"Did you feel your brother's presence?" Phil asked.

"Absolutely."

Phil asked me to recount the inhaling dream that had first made me aware of Tim. By then I had described it any number of times, but never before had my account of the dream been greeted with laughter. "Give her a chance," Phil told the audience.

"Later in the program," Phil said, "you'll meet other heart re-cipients who are at the very least scratching their heads over feelings that they have experienced, post-op, feelings they never had before, that lead them to wonder whether the central organ of the body, the heart muscle, when transplanted into another human being — whether somehow, accompanying this transfer, is a change of personality, interests, heretofore nonexistent. How do we explain this dream by Claire? Robert Bosnak, you're just who we're looking for."

Robbie: "What struck me most when I started to work with Claire was her tremendous drive and activity. What I couldn't explain was this tremendous drive, having to act constantly and do constantly."

Phil introduced the cardiac surgeon. "His team has per-formed over two hundred heart transplants," said Phil. "Does he buy this? What do you think? No! Well, here comes the grinch. Tell me how you think, you're the professional guy."

At least the surgeon wasn't hostile or rude. "If Claire inher-ited the kindness and the wonderful generosity of the donor family, that's great. But I don't think she inherited anything else, other than the heart."

This last remark was greeted by loud applause. Then Annie took him on: "How can you say that? How do you know how she feels? *You've* never had a heart transplant!"

Unknowingly, Annie had touched on one of the most com-mon complaints from the support groups I've been part of: that the doctors are usually quick to dismiss our reactions and feel-ings as illusory or unreal, although they themselves have never been in our situation. Moreover, most doctors and nurses don't even want to hear what we have to say.

The surgeon responded to Annie by saying, "The transplanted patients are terribly sick. Claire was an invalid, almost on her deathbed. The end of the line is there. She couldn't do anything more. Now, all of a sudden, we're putting a Corvette engine and lungs into almost a dead body, and the thing takes off and goes like crazy."

A viewer called in to say that before his heart transplant, he had always hated Italian food. After the operation, the first thing he asked for was linguine. He had a craving for spicy Italian food, and he learned later that his donor was Italian.

Somebody asked how I felt about motorcycles.

"I dislike them," I said, thinking of Kirk. "But a year after the transplant I had a love affair with a much younger man who rode motorcycles, and he had enormous energy, which seemed to match the energy in my heart. And he lived on the edge."

A woman asked if the people close to me felt that my personality had changed.

"My daughter is sitting right here," I replied. "And maybe she can answer."

Amara had been dreading this moment. Unlike her mother, she hates being the center of attention. I was enormously grateful that Amara had come with me and had agreed to sit in the audience. I was terribly nervous on that stage, but every time I glanced at Amara, who was smiling at me from the front row, she calmed me down. She had done me a great favor by coming on the show, and how was I repaying that kindness? By putting her on the spot. Thanks a lot, Mom!

Amara replied, as briefly as possible, that I had become more active and adventurous after the transplant.

A woman in the audience stood up to echo the surgeon's skepticism: "Of *course* she has more energy. She got a new heart! She got a second chance at life. Of course."

Then Robbie said, "There may be a last vestige of personality left in the heart. The motor of a Corvette — to use the doctor's analogy — has a different personality than the motor of a little car."

A few minutes later, Josie asked: "Why is it that the recipient can't know who the donor is? They should be given the choice. Why wasn't Claire allowed to know our name? It took a lot of courage for her to come to our house."

The surgeon said, "To encumber both families with the knowledge of these complex feelings becomes too difficult." In other words, Sorry, kids, Father knows best.

To which Josie replied, "I don't think that decision should be left up to the doctors and the hospitals. The families should make that decision!"

Near the end of the show, a woman stood up and said, "Traditional medicine is very limited. If something doesn't exist physically, it doesn't exist. When parts are taken from one person and moved to another person, we don't have the language for it in our vocabulary. But it's coming."

The next speaker was more direct: "I don't believe a damn word any of you are saying. I think you all need new brains!"

Phil: "I feel so much warm, positive energy!"

As the show ended, the surgeon was saying that the human heart was "nothing but a stupid pump."

I should have seen it coming. Although attitudes are definitely changing, we still live in an age where scientific, Western medicine is seen as the only valid truth. Now, there's a lot to be said for scientific, Western medicine, and nobody knows that better than I. Without it, I wouldn't be alive. But just because a phenomenon can't be explained by medical science doesn't mean it can't happen.

Some of the negative energy from the Donahue show reverberated for years. Gail, who watched it at home, was angry at me for implying, in her view, that it was easy and appropriate for transplant recipients to track down their donors. The next time we spoke, she shocked me by suggesting that I had seen Tim's obituary before calling her with his name — which made me so angry I hung up on her. For a long time we were out of touch, which was terribly difficult for both of us. I have always loved Gail, who had touched my heart both figuratively and literally, and I know that Gail loves me. We eventually resumed our friendship, and Gail apologized for what she said. But things have never been quite the same between us.

There was also a break with Tim's sisters. A couple of years later, after my third visit to Maine, they wrote that their family's relationship with me had become too painful, and they implied that I cared about them only as a source of information about my donor.

I was terribly upset when their letter arrived. Should I respond? Was it better to do nothing? I thought about it for weeks. I meditated on it, and spoke to my heart. It was almost as if I were asking Tim what I should do.

One morning, I focused on the image of a long-stemmed rose that I had seen the day before on a box of candy in a drugstore. Why a rose? Perhaps because in one of my dreams, the boy on a ship, who seemed to represent Tim, had given me a picture of a rose. And on the second Christmas after we met, June had sent me a blanket she had crocheted, which was decorated with pink and blue roses. I bought the candy and sent it to the parents of my heart with a simple note, saying that I was thinking of them with love and prayers.

A few days later, I was back at Yale for my annual exam, which always includes a heart catheterization and a biopsy. This is invariably a stressful time, because there's always a possibility that my heart or lungs are undergoing some form of rejection that I'm not even aware of. While I was there, Amara reached me to say that June had called to thank me for the candy, and to let me know I was always welcome in their home.

I was very moved, and June's message was even more welcome at this vulnerable time. I felt I had followed my heart and that Tim had wanted me to remain in touch. I still speak with June and Carl, but for now, at least, Tim's sisters and I are going our separate ways. My presence reminds them of a terribly painful event in their lives, and although I'm sad that we're not currently in touch, I can understand how they feel.

Sixteen

Moving On

WHILE MY connection to Tim is no longer as intense or as mystifying as it was before I met his family, three subsequent events have further illuminated the link between us. Oddly enough, two of them took place abroad.

First, a little background. Soon after I started working with Robbie, he suggested that I might want to experiment with choreographing various images from my dreams as another way of exploring them. The idea appealed to me, and with the help of another Jungian analyst who was also a dancer, I formed a small company called Dream Dancers. In 1991 I hosted a "Celebration of Life" party for transplant recipients and the hospital staff at Yale–New Haven Hospital, where our dance group performed a piece based on a composite of my various post-transplant dream images.

Around this time, Robbie began to organize what has since become an ongoing series of international conferences on dreams, where he brings together analysts, therapists, academics, artists, writers, policy makers, and other interested people from all over the world. Because dream choreography seemed to offer an exciting new approach, Robbie invited me to lead a workshop at the first of these gatherings, "Dreaming in Russia," which was held just outside Moscow in the summer of 1991. My workshop, which was one of many being offered at the conference, would include elements of dance, movement, meditation, music, and dreamwork. With participants attending from many different countries and speaking a variety of languages, there was a good deal of interest in a technique that explored the images and environments of dreams through movement, rather than words. The workshop was a success, and on the final night of the conference we performed some of our pieces for the entire group.

The whole conference was amazing, not only because it was the first meeting of its kind, but also because most of us who were coming from outside Russia happened to arrive in Moscow on the first day of the historic coup attempt of August 1991. Suddenly, the whole world was watching to see which way Russia would go — forward into freedom, or back, as the planners of the coup preferred, toward Russia's totalitarian past. Although the coup soon failed, for a few days we all experienced some anxious moments. I was feeling especially vulnerable, as I had brought along only enough cyclosporine for two weeks. As we watched, cut off from the rest of the world, the Russian people went through what seemed to me, at least, the political equivalent of a heart transplant. To their great joy, and ours, the operation succeeded with a minimum of rejection.

From the moment we landed in Russia, I had the sense of coming home. Seventy-eight years earlier, my grandparents had escaped from this troubled and violent land, together with their three-year-old daughter. They had left in search of political and religious freedom, and I felt privileged to be returning to Russia just as the very freedoms that my grandparents had yearned for were being recognized and valued.

How incredibly different this trip was from my visit to France the previous year. In France, all I had known about my heart was that it was inscrutable and apparently hyperactive. In France, Tim was returning to the land of *his* ancestors. In Russia, by contrast, I was leading my heart. I had to talk to my heart; I meditated to calm it down and get it in balance. The dramatic difference between these two trips seemed to epitomize my developing relationship with Tim: instead of identifying with the youthful spirit within me, I was now starting to integrate my new heart into my own personality and identity.

When the conference was over, my host family took me to see the sights of Moscow, where I was overwhelmed by a visit to a beautiful and ornate church. Inside that magnificent cathedral, with my Catholic heart beating strongly in my chest, I felt pulled to honor my donor. So I lit a candle for Tim, offered a silent prayer, and bought a set of amber beads for his mother. The entire time I was in that church, I experienced a powerful surge of love for Tim and his whole family. And I was grateful that their religious tradition, too, was a beneficiary of Russia's growing freedom.

The couple I stayed with in Moscow belonged to a large, extended family — like Tim's, in a way, and also like the family I had been part of long ago. Although my hosts, Zena and Armen, lived in a tiny, cramped apartment, they had strong, important relationships with a whole community of friends and relatives. And, just like my Russian grandparents, they also spoke naturally about their dreams. In fact, almost everything in their home — the lacy curtains, the vinyl tablecloth, the makeshift furniture — was reminiscent of my grandparents' apartment in the Bronx during the early 1950s.

When the time came to return to America, I didn't want to leave. After only a week with my hosts, I had become more attached than I realized. I felt a special warmth in Moscow, and a sense of connectedness. Suddenly my modest house on the ocean seemed like a huge indulgence. I was acutely aware of leaving a society where people had so little and shared so much, and returning to a place where people had so much and, all too often, shared so little.

Two years later, at a similar dream conference in Greece, I experienced another emotional link to Tim. Soon after I arrived, one of the participants introduced me to an American couple in their fifties. Their son had died two years ago, and they had donated his organs. But they didn't seem eager to talk about it, and I didn't press them.

The next morning, the father showed up at my dream choreography workshop. He was sitting next to me, and when his assigned workshop partner abruptly left him to team up with someone else, he turned toward me. As the leader, I was available to help anyone who needed a partner, so the two of us began working together. Within minutes, this man was initiating a series of silent gestures that involved giving and taking from one heart to another. Because I knew his story, I could see that he, as the donor, was offering up the organs of his son. I, as the recipient, began accepting them, as we symbolically ritualized the process of donating and receiving the organs of life. It was clear that both his movements and mine were coming from a deep place within each of us.

Later, when the session was over, the participants in the workshop were offered the opportunity to show their pieces to the rest of the group. To my surprise, my partner, who seemed to cherish his privacy, was eager to share what we had done.

Our performance was even more emotional the second time, and we expanded it into a longer piece. When we were finished, we collapsed, sobbing, into each other's arms. Although the other participants didn't know the literal story we were acting out, they were transfixed.

The next day, a close friend of this man told me that this was the first time the father had been able to grieve for his son. But I wondered if he knew that this ritual had been just as important for me. Although the father of my own heart was thousands of miles away, I felt that I was going through these movements not only for myself, but also for Carl, as if this performance could in some way help him repair his relationship with his deceased son.

And maybe, somehow, it did. The fractured connection between Carl and Tim had been tugging at me ever since my first visit to Maine. Father's Day had come along a few days later, and when I found myself in a card shop I bought a beautiful card for Carl. But I never mailed it — not only because it felt presumptuous, but also because I had the feeling that Tim wouldn't have sent his father a card — at least not at that stage of their relationship.

Months after the conference in Greece, when I returned to Maine to visit Tim's parents, I noticed a real difference in Carl's reaction to me. He smiled, he was outgoing, and I felt that we were becoming friends. He gave me a flower from his garden, and he tugged at my heart when he said, "You are part of our family now."

Later that day, at Tim's grave, Carl said, "You know, June, something's going on up there. Doesn't Claire remind you of my sister, especially her eyes?"

June laughed. But it was clear to me that Carl was feeling the connection between us. Somehow, since my previous visit, some healing and reconciliation had occurred between father and son.

Each year, when the anniversary of my transplant rolls around, I have dreams that feel especially significant. On the first anniversary of my new life, I dreamed that my mother came to me and placed a large gold amulet on my chest. The second year, I dreamed about a horrible noise that was reminiscent of a surgical saw slicing through skin. On my third anniversary, I saw myself floating in space, covered in white, and shaking, as if my heart had just been shocked back into life — as it had been during the transplant.

In 1992, on my fourth anniversary, I dreamed that I was revving up twenty-two motorcycles that I was supposed to drive around town to commemorate something — but I didn't know what. The motorcycles seemed to be an obvious reference to Tim, but why, I wondered, where there twenty-two of them? Was there any special significance to that number? Then it hit me: this was the fourth anniversary of the transplant, which meant that Tim, had he lived, would now be twenty-two.

This dream seemed to be calling me to reenact Tim's great passion — riding a motorcycle. I called a friend, a dancer who owns a motorcycle, and on the last Saturday night in May the two of us went out dancing. I was wearing an evening dance dress, high heels, and a motorcycle helmet, and as the sun was setting over the Charles River, he drove me at full speed from one dance to another. My heart was exhilarated to be zipping along like this, although the rest of me, frankly, found the experience a little frightening.

As the evening went on, I seemed to be enjoying myself less and less. Something was changing, and although I didn't realize this at the time, I now believe that ritualizing the motorcycle dream allowed me to gently release Tim's spirit. I had finally achieved my new identity, a kind of third being that was neither the old Claire nor the new Tim, but some combination of the two.

It was no accident, I believe, that soon after this evening I was able to welcome a new man into my life in a more permanent way. It was as if Tim had stepped aside, leaving room in my heart for somebody else.

Ever since the transplant, I have been interested in ballroom dancing. I love it all, from the costumes to the intricate foot-work, and I enjoy the fact that my fellow dancers are a truly diverse group. They are amateurs in the best sense of the word: they love dancing and they do it for pleasure.

It was at a dance that I mct Jerry, my new companion. Al-though we come from very different backgrounds and outlooks, for the past few years we have been partners both in life and in dance. We often enter competitions together, competing in both "smooth" (fox-trot, waltz, Viennese waltz, and tango) and "Latin" (swing, cha-cha, mambo, rumba, and merengue). And partly through our dancing, Jerry has brought me back into my body, back toward the earth.

Does Jerry, too, have a connection with Tim? I wouldn't have thought so, but life is full of surprises. When I first met Jerry, he was involved with a woman named Cindy. Later on, when Jerry and I were together, we were celebrating my birthday when he suddenly realized that July 29 was also Cindy's birthday. Later that evening, he overheard me telling someone that my donor had come from Milford, Maine.

"Milford?" said Jerry. "Did you say Milford?"

"Yes, why?"

"That's where Cindy comes from. We used to drive up there to visit her family. I did a few outreach programs at a church in Milford with some of the teenagers."

If this were a novel, Jerry and Tim would have known each other. But Tim's name didn't ring a bell. Maybe it's enough that Jerry was involved with two women who were born on the same day. And that one of these women came from the same little town as the young man whose heart and lungs were keeping the other woman alive.

Seventeen

Other Voices

FOR YEARS, Robbie and I have wondered whether the kinds of things that have happened to me have also happened, in one way or another, to a significant number of other heart recipients. If our New Haven research group is any guide, the answer may be yes. On the other hand, our sample was too small and self-selected to suggest any larger implications.

It sounds like a simple question, but it's not. For one thing, although hospital policies are beginning to change, most transplant recipients know little or nothing about their donors. For another, those people who do experience puzzling or provocative dreams, or who notice surprising or inexplicable changes in their lives, are generally reluctant to talk about it. After all, nobody enjoys being thought of as a kook. The doctors and nurses who care for transplant recipients are generally skeptical, dismissive, or even contemptuous of such testimonies, which are typically seen as being caused by the powerful medications that all of us must take. When a recipient asks about a puzzling personal change, he or she is often told, as I was, "Don't worry about it. Get on your exercise bike."

Another obstacle to investigating this question is the almost inevitable occurrence of denial, which appears to be common among heart-transplant patients. In the early 1980s, Dr. François Mai, a Canadian psychiatrist, interviewed twenty new heart recipients within three months of their transplants. "The most striking finding," he reported, "was the presence of denial in 18 of the 20 patients (90%)." As examples of denial, he cited such statements as "I've no feelings about having a new heart," and "I never think about the donor."

Dr. Mai, it should be noted, was referring to basic feelings and curiosity about the transplant or the donor, rather than unusual or mysterious occurrences. He also suggested that such denial, at least in the early stages of a patient's recovery, may serve an important protective and adaptive function. "It is not surprising," he concluded, "that feelings of anxiety, conflict, and ambivalence were present and only thinly disguised. Denial may be seen as a means of coping with, or perhaps of postponing these feelings until they could be better accommodated."*

In another study, a cardiac surgeon reported that one of his patients, a used-car dealer, seemed to be showing no anxiety about his recent heart transplant. A week after the operation, the surgeon showed the patient his old heart, which was preserved in a jar of formaldehyde.

"Doesn't it make you feel a little odd looking at your heart?" the surgeon asked. "Don't you have some sort of emotional tie to it?"

Apparently not. "I've owned a lot of cars in my life," the patient replied. "Not one of them did I develop an emotional attachment to."†

---

* François M. Mai, M.D., "Graft and Donor Denial in Heart Transplant Recipients," *American Journal of Psychiatry,* vol. 143, no. 9 (September 1986), pp. 1159–1161; p. 1161.

† Quoted in Pietro Castelnuovo-Tedesco, "Cardiac Surgeons Look at Transplantation," *Seminars in Psychiatry,* vol. 3, no. 1 (February 1971), pp. 5–16; p. 7. I especially like this story because it reverses the stereotype: here the surgeon is surprised that the patient is emotionally uninvolved.

This, of course, may be an extreme example of denial. But if heart transplant recipients typically repress even a mild curiosity about their donors, they would be even more likely to avoid any thoughts or feelings they might have about taking on some aspects of the donor's spirit. For many people, the idea of carrying another presence inside is so threatening, and so utterly preposterous, that one common response, surely, would be to repress or deny it completely. At the same time, the likelihood that such feelings would be repressed or denied certainly doesn't prove that the recipients ever felt them in the first place.

There is also *conscious* denial. A year or two after their transplants, many recipients prefer to look forward, not back. The period following a transplant is often a painful and difficult one, and even if some events during that time were difficult to understand, recipients often choose to focus instead on their new lives.

Another, very different concern is also part of this skeptical mix. Among both recipients and transplant professionals, I have found a real and understandable fear that any public discussion of this controversial and potentially disturbing topic might exacerbate an already-serious problem. Ever since human organ transplants began, a severe shortage of donors has led to thousands of preventable deaths each year. While I don't believe that a public airing of these issues will scare off potential organ donors, I certainly understand this concern. So let me be clear: organ donation really *is* the gift of life, and nothing I have said or speculated about in these pages is meant to obscure or dilute this important truth.

Despite all the reasons that make it difficult to document unusual occurrences among transplant recipients, at least one researcher has collected quite a few of them. Dr. Paul Pearsall, a neuropsychologist at Wayne State University School of Medicine and a bestselling author and lecturer who underwent a bone marrow transplant in 1987, is writing a book whose working title is *Cellular Memories: The New Psychology of the Heart.* When I spoke with Dr. Pearsall in early 1997, he had gathered more than seventy personal testimonies from transplant recipients whose experiences cannot easily be explained by contemporary Western medicine.

Dr. Pearsall's interest in this subject began after his own transplant. A fellow patient, who was also undergoing a bone marrow transplant, insisted that he could feel the presence of his donor. Dr. Pearsall asked the man what he thought his donor was like.

"Some kind of artist," he replied. "Maybe a painter or a musician."

Later, the patient was informed that his donor's hobby was oil painting.

Following a recent lecture on the unusual experiences reported by transplant recipients, Dr. Pearsall was challenged by an orthopedic surgeon in the audience. Some recipients, said the surgeon, may *need* to tell these stories, which, he added, are invariably fabricated, even when the patient sincerely believes that such things actually happened.

"If these patients 'need' to make up stories," Dr. Pearsall replied, "they seem awfully reluctant to talk about them. They are as bothered and amazed by these experiences as anyone. As a transplant recipient myself, I may be a little more willing to listen to the story rather than doubting the teller. As a doctor, I usually talk too much and listen too little anyway."

When we spoke, Dr. Pearsall referred to me and the other transplant recipients he had interviewed as "white crows" — a reference to the psychologist William James, who wrote that in order to disprove the law that all crows are black, it is enough to produce a single white crow. Dr. Pearsall believes that the existence of these "white crows" requires a whole new set of explanations, which will, I hope, be explored in his book.

When Robert Bosnak and I interviewed transplant recipients, we, too, found that most of them were not especially eager to discuss their unusual experiences. In most cases, the people we spoke with asked us not to use their real names, and we honored that request. The day will come, I expect, when cases like mine will be studied in a systematic way. Until then, we will have to make do with anecdotal evidence.

A transplant nurse in Florida told us about a heart-transplant patient who, before her operation, had suffered from an extreme fear of water — a fear so debilitating that she wouldn't even take a shower. Soon after her transplant, this same woman felt a great desire to go swimming and sailing. A surgical resident, who wasn't authorized to disclose this information, informed the woman's incredulous family that her donor had been an avid sailor who died in a boating accident.

This same nurse also told us about a middle-aged man who received a new heart from a young donor who was killed in a motorcycle accident. The recipient, a born-again Christian, woke up from the operation cursing and swearing, which was completely out of character. Because the donor had died at the same hospital where the transplant was performed, the donor's mother ended up meeting the recipient. She confirmed that the man was speaking just like her son, and was even using some of the same mannerisms.

If our informal survey is any indication, the most commonly noticed changes reported by transplant recipients have to do with new food preferences. This seems to be especially common among recipients who have received a new kidney: a

Michigan man who never liked coffee received a kidney from his sister, a big coffee drinker; soon he, too, was drinking coffee. A woman who donated a kidney to her husband reported that he now craves what used to be her favorite foods. She still enjoys them, but now that one of her kidneys is gone, she no longer *loves* these foods. We heard many such stories among both kidney and heart recipients — the steak-eater who became a vegetarian; the milk-drinker who began to hate milk; the man who always wanted to like wine, but never enjoyed it until after his transplant. The number and the persistence of these accounts seem to suggest that food preferences may be based not only in the mind or the taste buds, but may have some deeper biological roots.

The most amazing case we heard about is the man who actually ran a race against his old heart. It sounds impossible, but this is how it happened. Mr. A., a patient in England, was suffering from cystic fibrosis; although he needed a new pair of lungs, his heart was strong. He received a heart-lung transplant, whereupon his old but still-healthy heart was removed and implanted into the body of Mr. B., whose own heart was failing. (This type of procedure, which doesn't happen often, is known as a "domino" transplant.)

In 1994, at the annual Transplant Games in England, Mr. A. had the singular experience, surely unparalleled in human history, of racing against his old heart — which, from its new location in Mr. B.'s chest, outran its former owner. After the race, the two men sat down and talked together. Mr. B. told Mr. A. about his new food cravings, and Mr. A. confirmed that these were also *his* favorites. (Whether they were *still* Mr. A.'s favorite foods, now that he no longer had his original heart, is not clear.)*

* The story of the two runners appears in Daniel Jeffreys, "Have These Transplant Patients Inherited the Donor's Characters?" London *Daily Mail,* June 4, 1996, p. 51.

In New Mexico, a young recipient received the heart and lungs of a girl who had been chased and murdered by members of an Asian gang. Although the murder hadn't yet been announced, when the young man awoke from the operation he described a vision he'd had of a blond girl being chased down the street by small, slightly built men who wanted to kill her. Later, the girl's mother discussed this incident on a television talk show. One of the recipient's nurses wrote about it in the Buddhist magazine *Tricycle,* and wondered if this incident might lend credence to theories about "cellular memory."

Harriet, a physician, was one of Paul Pearsall's patients. Years ago, on a rainy night, she and her husband were driving home from a party. They'd had an argument, and now they were riding in silence. The only sound in their car was the persistent clicking of the windshield wipers. Suddenly, out of nowhere, another car came crashing through their windshield. Harriet was knocked unconscious; her husband was killed.

He had signed an organ donor card, and when Harriet awoke in the hospital, she weakly gave permission for his heart to be donated. Years after this event, she came to Dr. Pearsall for help. She had tried everything, she told him, including psychics and mediums, in an effort to make contact with her deceased husband. She asked Dr. Pearsall if it might be possible for her to meet the young man who received her husband's heart. "I want to feel that heart again," she told him. "I know this sounds crazy, but I can't help it."

After many calls and conversations, Pearsall was able to arrange a meeting between Harriet and the recipient of her husband's heart. As Pearsall and Harriet waited for the young man to arrive, Harriet suddenly said, "He's here. I can feel him." The recipient, who was coming with his mother, wasn't expected for another half hour. But a moment later, the young man walked into the room.

"Can I hold you?" Harriet asked him. For several moments they stood chest to chest, crying. Later, Harriet asked if she could feel his heart. The young man nodded and placed her hand against his naked chest. "I love you, sweetie," she said. Then she slowly removed her hand. The young man put on his shirt and nodded again, as if to indicate that he understood to whom this comment was directed.

"I felt him," Harriet said softly. "I could almost hear him. Not his voice, but him. I could feel his essence, his energy. I know it's okay now."

The young man began to giggle. "I'm sorry," he said, "but I suddenly feel lighthearted. For the first time, my heart actually feels light."

His mother, who hadn't said much, suddenly spoke up: "That's the one thing the doctors couldn't explain. My son has always said that his new heart was too heavy in his chest. The doctors assured him it was all in his mind, but he kept saying it was too heavy."

"It isn't anymore," her son said. "It feels like it just got opened up, or cleared out."

He and Harriet talked a little more, and discussed several changes in the recipient that seemed to correlate with Harriet's husband. Then, just before he left, the young man turned to Harriet and said, "You know, there's just one thing I don't understand. Ever since the transplant, I've been bothered by the clicking of the windshield wipers on my car. I don't suppose you would know what *that's* about?"

Eighteen

Searching
for Answers

"I CAN'T BLAME you for feeling this way," a doctor told me not long ago. "If I were carrying somebody else's heart and lungs within me, I'd probably have all kinds of thoughts and fantasies about the donor. For centuries, poets and artists have told us that the heart is a great repository of spirit and emotion. That's a beautiful idea, but clinically there's nothing to it. The heart is just a pump."

This, of course, is the view of contemporary Western medicine. I say "contemporary" because until the seventeenth century, the heart wasn't seen as a pump at all. In antiquity, it was regarded as the center of wisdom and emotion. In some ancient societies, victorious warriors would eat the hearts of their vanquished enemies in order to acquire their strength. In the Hebrew Bible, where the word *lev* (heart) occurs more than a thousand times, the heart was seen as the center of both knowledge and morality. Aristotle believed the heart was the center of thought and sensation. In the Middle Ages, kings and prominent clergymen would arrange for their bodies to be buried in one graveyard and their hearts in another.

In 1648, in one of the most significant discoveries in the history of medicine, the English physician William Harvey proclaimed to the world that the heart, through a continual series of contractions, pumps blood throughout the body and returns it to its source. Today, of course, nobody argues this point. But to acknowledge what is now obvious — that the heart *is* a pump — is not the same as insisting that it is *only* a pump. As we'll see, some scientists believe that the heart may actually be a good deal more.

At this point, frankly, I am out of my element. While I can speak with confidence about the precise nature of my own experiences, when it comes to explaining these events I have no special knowledge or expertise. While I seem to have inherited some aspects of Tim's spirit and personality, I don't pretend to know how this happened.

But because I'm too curious to let it go at that, I have asked several open-minded scientists, authors, and other experts how they would account for my experience. A number of respondents used the phrase "cellular memory," although they seemed to be divided as to exactly what the term means, and whether it should be regarded as fact or theory. This phrase, incidentally, was originally used with regard to the immune system; decades after receiving a polio vaccine, for example, our bodies still retain a "memory" of that particular antigen.

Deepak Chopra is among those who seem to assume an enhanced understanding of cellular memory. In one of his popular books, he reports that some transplant patients, after receiving a new kidney, liver, or heart, begin to participate in their donors' memories. As he puts it, "Associations that belonged to another person start being released when that person's tissues are placed inside a stranger." After describing my own case, Chopra offers this interpretation:

Rather than seeking a supernatural explanation for such in-
cidents, one could see them as confirmation that our bodies
are made of experiences transformed into physical expression. Because experience is something we incorporate (literally, "make into a body"), our cells have been instilled
with our memories; thus, to receive someone else's cells is
to receive their memories at the same time.*

While many scientists do not accept the idea of cellular
memory, a growing number now believe that every cell in our
body has its own "mind." Some go further, and postulate that if
you transfer tissues from one body to another, the cells from the
first body will carry memories into the second body.

But what kinds of memories can exist in human organs? Like
most people, I used to assume that all of our intelligence was
concentrated in the brain. But that was before I learned about
the work of Candace Pert, the biochemist who discovered that
at least one aspect of our minds was distributed throughout our
bodies. Pert found that the brain and the body communicate
with each other through short chains of amino acids known as
neuropeptides and receptors. Human emotions, says Pert, are
triggered by neuropeptides attaching themselves to receptors,
which stimulates an electrical change in neurons.

While peptides were known to exist in the brain, Pert and
her colleagues have found them throughout the body, including
the heart. There are even neuropeptides in our stomachs,
which, I suppose, gives a whole new meaning to the expression
"gut feeling."

Dozens of these peptides have now been identified, and each

* Deepak Chopra, *Ageless Body, Timeless Mind* (New York, 1993), p. 23.

has its own type of receptor. Receptors, which are situated on the surface of the cell, are often compared to locks, with the neuropeptides functioning as keys. Unless the right key is applied to the appropriate lock, nothing happens.

When Pert first began her research, she, too, assumed that the mind and the emotions were located in the brain. Now, she says, she can no longer make a strong distinction between body and mind.

I asked Bruce Lipton, a former Stanford research scientist who was trained in cellular and developmental biology, how Pert's ideas might apply to transplant recipients:

> A transplanted heart comes with the donor's unique set of self-receptors, which differ, naturally, from those of the recipient. As a result, the recipient now possesses cells which respond to two different "identities." Not every recipient will sense that a set of cells within their body is now responding to a second signal. But if anyone is going to experience this change, it might well be a dancer who is acutely aware of her own body. As more and more transplants are performed, I think we'll see a growing number of people reporting these experiences.
>
> Here's another way to look at it. You're listening to a portable radio, and the batteries go dead. Did the broadcast stop? Of course not. You can put in new batteries, or you can get another radio and tune it to the same station. Our biological bodies are like cellular radios, and each of our cells is tuned to the same station through our molecular antennae. Our identities are the stations, and even if we die, if our cells are still tuned to our station, they'll still play it — even if those cells are now in another person's body.

Bruce Lipton urged me to contact Cleve Backster, and I did. Backster, a pioneer in the development and application of lie detectors, first came to public attention in the 1960s, when his experiments suggested that plants could communicate with other forms of life on a cellular level, and could even experience what appeared to be the botanical equivalent of certain human emotions.

These days, Backster performs experiments with human cells, which lead him to believe that leukocytes (white blood cells) can communicate with each other *even when some of these cells have been separated from the rest of the body*. In a series of experiments, Backster has removed white cells from the mouths of volunteers. These cells are then centrifuged — separated out with a kind of high-speed spin dryer — placed in a test tube, and hooked up to a kind of electroencephalograph, which is normally used to monitor brain waves. Backster has found that when the donor is subjected to certain emotional stimuli, such as fear, excitement, or anger, there is usually an unmistakable reaction from the separated cells, even if they are miles away.

I asked Backster whether these findings had any implications for transplant recipients.

"The only cells I've worked with," he replied, "come from the gums and the roof of the mouth. If we can project onto heart cells, then some form of communication might still exist with the cells of the donors — except for the fact that the donor is dead. I've been able to show that separated cells can communicate with the cells of live donors. Can they also communicate with the cells of dead donors? I don't know the answer. At that point you'd be getting into metaphysics, which is a whole other discussion."

Julie Motz, whose work has been featured on NBC's *Dateline* and in *The New York Times Magazine,* is an "energy healer" who has participated in open-heart surgeries and heart-transplant operations at Columbia-Presbyterian Medical Center in New York. At first she worked with patients before and after their surgeries, preparing their minds and bodies for the operation, and helping them when the surgery was over. Eventually she became curious as to whether she could also be effective within the operating room:

> As a healer, much of my work involves uncovering the emotional states which accompany physical conditions, and helping my clients to experience them. I had long been aware that the body appeared to hold memories in different areas, and that these could be released through energy and touch. From Bonnie Bainbridge Cohen in Massachusetts, I learned that each cell in the body acts like a brain and can be consciously addressed.
>
> Sometimes our tissues carry the energy of specific emotions which have not been consciously processed. For example, when I ask heart transplant patients to go down inside their bodies and "be their blood," a feeling of sadness often comes to me in my own blood, which I believe is picking up a sympathetic vibration from theirs. Later, when I ask these patients to allow their blood to thank their old heart for all it has done for them, and to lovingly say goodbye to it, the sadness gradually eases.
>
> Claire, I believe that the cells of the organs that were transplanted into you had memory, including both ideation and emotion. These memories were communicated to the other cells in your body, including your nervous system, which then picked up these messages and sent them to your

brain. Your brain, acting like a tuner or receiver, then turned them into conscious memory.

Like Julie Motz, Paul Pearsall, the neuropsychologist who is writing a book about heart recipients, also speaks in terms of the energy that exists in our bodies:

Anyone who receives a new heart is getting a big ball of subtle energy. Ancient cultures have known about subtle energy throughout history, and have viewed it as the vital force of all creation. The indigenous peoples of the world have more than a hundred different names for this force, and unlike us, they have always placed their faith in its power. The Chinese call it *chi*. The Japanese call it *ki*. In Hawaii it's known as *Mana*. Mana is the spirit of life itself, and the place where memories are stored. No matter how materialistic our modern world has become, something keeps tugging at our hearts and drawing us back to the energy that brings us life, unites us in love, and leaves our physical body when we die. Physicists call this energy "the fifth force." It's the same energy that keeps messing up the "controlled" experiments of scientists and accounts for "spontaneous remissions" in so-called terminal cases.

I don't have much doubt about cellular memory. The more interesting question, at least to me, is, Why do some people have these experiences, and not others? What I've learned from the dozens of organ recipients I've interviewed is that the individuals who feel these changes are unusually aware of their bodies. They're often artists, painters, or poets — creative people, in other words, who are introspective and paying attention.

Pearsall offers an intriguing response to those who wonder if the unusual experiences of some transplant recipients might be a result of the potent antirejection medications that we all must take:

> I don't doubt for a moment that the lethal substances we pump into these people can have powerful psychological effects. But maybe there's another way to understand this psychopharmacology. Why are these stories so consistent? Why do recipients have the memories of a donor they never knew, and whom we can sometimes identify? Maybe these drugs act like LSD or some other hallucinogenic agent, and enhance perception in a way that helps us look where we never looked before. Is it not possible that our immuno-suppressant drugs are somehow lowering our patients' thresholds for accessibility to the cellular memories we all have?

Paul Pearsall referred me to the HeartMath Institute in Boulder Creek, California, where researchers are studying the energy of the heart as well as the connection and possible communication between the heart and the brain. Rollin McCraty is the institute's research director. "Your experiences are not unique," he told me:

> A number of physicians come to our institute, and over the years I've heard other stories like this. One cardiac surgeon told me that he has observed this phenomenon, which includes personality changes and cravings for new foods, and that it usually fades a few months after the transplant. It's not something surgeons want publicized, and they keep it very quiet.
> We know, from recent research, that the heart is a far

more intelligent organ than we thought. It now appears that the heart has its own intrinsic nervous system, which Dr. Andrew Armour, the author of *Neurocardiology*, calls "the little brain in the heart."

Another possible clue might come from a recent discovery in Boston. In 1995, Dr. Ming-He Huang, a Harvard Medical School researcher, discovered a new type of cell in the heart. These "intrinsic cardiac adrenergic" (ICA) cells seem to synthesize and release catecholamines — a group name for a bunch of different chemicals, like dopamine, which used to be thought of as exclusive to the brain. ICA cells have magnetic properties, which suggests that the heart can respond to and interact with magnetic fields. A similar type of magnetic cell can be found in the brain. There may well be an electro-magnetic connection between the heart and the brain, and the discovery of these new cells seems to support that possibility.

Gary E. Schwartz, Ph.D., is professor of psychology, neurology, and psychiatry, and director of the Human Energy Systems Laboratory at the University of Arizona. Schwartz and his colleague, Dr. Linda G. Russek, have proposed a mathematical explanation for how everything in nature, including all cellular and molecular systems, stores information and energy. Their theory, which they call the Systemic Memory hypothesis, is too complex to summarize here even if I could. It provides a new explanation for, among other phenomena, memory from organ transplants (cellular memory); homeopathy (memory in water); and psychometry (memory in objects):

Systemic memory predicts that all transplant patients register stored information and energy from the donor's tissues — certainly unconsciously, and sometimes consciously. In our view, the problem of organ rejection involves not only the rejection of the material of the cells, but also the information and energy stored within the cells and molecules.

You received a large amount of core tissue — the heart and the lungs, which can store substantial information and energy. You are also a dancer, in touch with your body. Finally, you're emotionally sensitive and open to spiritual information. You were primed, then, to resonate with all of this information and energy, not only unconsciously, but consciously as well. It may well be that because you accepted your donor's information and energy, you were better able to accept and incorporate the new heart and lungs. This could explain why you've had so few problems with rejection over the years, and why you're thriving today.

We have also published research showing that the heart and brain communicate with each other both energetically and physiologically. Specifically, the heart's electrocardiogram can be registered in our brain waves. Moreover, loving people can register, in their brain waves, the electrocardiograms of other people's hearts. This research provides a biophysical explanation for how a transplant recipient could register the energy and information coming from her new heart and lungs.

People speak of learning things "by heart." Is this simply a misplaced metaphor, or could there be some deeper significance to this phrase? If all cells store information and energy, and if the heart is especially involved in this process because of the centrality of its location and connections, then memories — especially implicit memories — may literally involve the heart as well as the brain. And if a heart is transplanted, some aspects of the donor's history will potentially be accessible to the recipient.

At this point in our discussion we leave the world of material reality to consider several other ways of understanding what happened to me.

For James Van Praagh, a spiritual medium in Los Angeles, my experience was caused by a spirit that hadn't yet moved on to its next home:

> Donated organs often come from young people who were killed in car or motorcycle accidents, and who died quickly. Because their spirits often feel they haven't completed their time on earth, they sometimes attach themselves to another person. There may be things that your donor hadn't completed in the physical world, which his spirit still wanted to experience. When this happens, the spirit is caught between two worlds, like in the movie *Ghost*. Sometimes this leads to possession, and sometimes, as in your case, to influences. If this is what happened, I expect that Tim's spirit will eventually move on when he realizes that he no longer needs to experience the physical world. Perhaps this has already happened.
>
> Dreams are often communications with spirits. The easiest way for spirits to communicate with us is when we're not in our daytime, rational minds. When you had those dreams, Tim's spirit was working with you.

Rupert Sheldrake, an English scientist, is the author of several fascinating books, including *Seven Experiments That Could Change the World* and *The Presence of the Past,* which explores the idea of "morphic resonance" — the transmission of forms and behaviors through repetition in time. Sheldrake questions the accepted idea that memories are stored inside our heads. Our minds, he suggests, may be more like television sets than video recorders; a television tunes in to transmissions, but it doesn't store them.

In a letter commenting on my experience, Sheldrake notes that my story reminds him of cases of reincarnation and reports of past lives. He then suggests two other possibilities:

> I don't know what to make of the dreams and memories that Claire Sylvia experienced as evidence of transmitted memory. Even if she knew things about the young man which she could not have known normally, there is the possibility that she picked up this information telepathically from people at the hospital. This would not, however, explain her cravings for beer and chicken nuggets.
>
> If there is indeed a transmission of memory through the heart and lungs, I would not attribute it to cellular memory. However impressive this may sound, it has no basis in current science and there is no known way in which cells could store psychological memories. The current materialistic theories of science would locate these memories in the brain, not in the heart and lungs.
>
> My own hypothesis, which is also beyond the limits of conventional science, would perhaps permit a transfer of memories without requiring it to be embedded inside the cells *per se*. This explanation, which is developed in detail in *The Presence of the Past*, allows for memory transfer between individuals and between generations. From this point of view, the heart and lungs of the young man would be associated with his morphic fields. These could then be experi-

enced by Claire Sylvia. But this transfer of memory need
not depend on physical traces within the cells.

Sheldrake's mention of reincarnation and past lives leads naturally to the work of Brian Weiss, the author of *Many Lives, Many
Masters* and *Only Love Is Real*. I was surprised, therefore, that Dr.
Weiss's interpretation of my experience did not draw upon his
interest in past lives, but referred instead to the practice of psychometry. Psychometry, which is also known as object reading,
is the ability of some people to pick up mental images of another person simply by holding an object that belongs to them:

> If it's possible to pick up impressions from holding some-
> body's watch, imagine what it must be like to receive or-
> gans that have been imbued for years with another person's
> energy. So it doesn't surprise me that you can tap into this
> young man's emotions, preferences, and inclinations. I see
> your experience as a psychic phenomenon having to do
> with energy rather than, say, possession. People have differ-
> ing levels of psychic awareness, and some organ recipients
> might well be sensitive to their donor's energy.
>
> It may also be no accident that you were the recipient
> who ended up with these organs. Perhaps there was some
> other connection between you and Tim, either in the
> present or in the past, that has yet to be uncovered.

Larry Dossey, who offers several possible explanations, is a
physician of internal medicine and the author of, among other
books, *Recovering the Soul* and *Healing Words: The Power of Prayer
and the Practice of Medicine*. He is also executive editor of the
journal *Alternative Therapies in Health and Medicine*.

The possibility that a living person might take on the personality traits, behaviors, and even memories of a deceased individual is an ancient concept. This is the idea behind reincarnation, the belief that there is a continuity between individuals living and dead.

Can donated organs mediate such a continuity? And if so, how? The biologist Lyall Watson, in his book *The Nature of Things: The Secret Life of Inanimate Objects,* proposes that physical items with which we are in intimate contact can somehow take on our "emotional fingerprints" and store our thoughts and feelings. Later, under the right conditions, they can come to life, as it were, and act in surprisingly lifelike ways. Watson has collected a vast array of examples suggesting such an effect — cars starting up by themselves and driving off, for example, and objects such as rings, jewelry, and dolls that behave as if they were alive.

If inanimate objects can store our feelings and thoughts, why not our own body parts? But how this might happen is not clear.

Far more likely, in my view, is that the consciousness of the donor is fundamentally united with the consciousness of the recipient, which enabled you to gain information about your donor. Receiving the donor's heart did not actually cause a mechanical transfer of experiences from one person to another, but somehow intensified a mental connection that was already present.

Surveys show that most people experience, at least occasionally, phenomena such as telepathy, clairvoyance, and precognition. And many of us have experiences suggesting that our minds are indeed united. Some of the strongest evidence for this comes from studies in distant healing and prayer. In a 1988 experiment, Dr. Randolph Byrd examined the effects of intercessory prayer in about 400 heart patients in the coronary care unit at San Francisco General Hospital. Half of the patients received prayer, while the other half did not. This was a double-blind study, meaning that no one involved in the experiment knew who was, or wasn't, receiving prayer. When the study was concluded, those patients who received distant prayer did better, on average, than those who didn't.

We are gradually arriving at a picture of consciousness that I call *nonlocal mind* — what our ancestors called the Universal Mind, or the One Mind. In this view, the mind is not limited by time or space; it cannot be localized or confined to individual brains and bodies, or even to the present. At some dimension of consciousness we are all united as a single, seamless whole. But most of us prefer to retain the idea that we are solitary individuals, isolated physically and mentally from everyone else.

Throughout history, however, people have discovered ways of realizing their mental connections with others. Sometimes physical objects serve this purpose, as in a ring that helps two lovers realize their unity. Both parties understand that the ring doesn't contain their actual memories and thoughts, and that it's a symbol that triggers associations in the consciousness of the people involved. Could a part of the body, such as a donated heart or kidney, function symbolically in a similar way?

Consider palm-reading. The person whose palm is read is temporarily "donating" his hand to the palm reader, the "recipient," who uses the palm to make a mental connection with the individual who is seeking information. Some palm readers acknowledge that the palm is merely a device, a go-between that allows the palmist to enter that realm of consciousness where information about another person can be accessed. I wonder: could the heart that you received have been functioning as a palm, enabling you to focus attention in a dimension that would normally be closed to you, and to gain information about your donor?

I also wonder: are other organ recipients having similar experiences? Before it became acceptable to speak of them, we believed that near-death experiences were rare. But when people who underwent resuscitation in modern hospitals were surveyed, it turned out that these experiences were actually rather common. Post-transplant experiences such as yours may also be more widespread than we think.

I find it both exciting and gratifying that scientists and other thinkers have so many ideas and explanations for the things that have happened to me. I am fascinated by the research of Candace Pert, which seems to be breaking down the old and often artificial walls between body and mind. I am amazed by the experiments of Cleve Backster, which appear to show that our cells are somehow linked together even when they are physically separated. Brian Weiss's analogy to psychometry strikes me as a real possibility, while Paul Pearsall's speculations on the possible effects of antirejection medication are fascinating.

To be sure, the interpretations offered in this chapter do not come out of conventional science or medicine. Many of the experts quoted here operate well outside the mainstream, and a few of their comments and conjectures may strike readers as far-fetched or even absurd. That's because some of them probably *are* absurd.

But which ones? When Harvey announced that the heart was

a pump, many of his colleagues thought *that* was absurd. When you invite intelligent, creative people to speculate about mysterious events that are entirely new in human history, the ensuing conversation will cover a wide spectrum of possibilities. This discussion is just beginning.

A Final Word

MY JOURNEY continues, although in the telling it inevitably becomes a slightly different story from the one I am living. In the reading, it will probably become slightly different again, in much the same way a dancer brings her own experience and feelings to someone else's choreography.

I sometimes wonder whether my entire earlier life was a preparation for the transplant and its aftermath. The family I was raised in, my rebelliousness, my dancing, my illnesses, my immersion in alternative medicine, my interest in dreams — by the time Tim's spirit merged with mine, I was already prepared and open to receive his strengthening energy. I have always believed in the power of the mind and the emotions, and in realities that are not necessarily visible and concrete.

Although Tim's life was cut short, his spirit, along with his organs, were evidently meant to continue living. I believe, as Tim's mother does, that he led me to find his family, to be in touch with them again, and perhaps to resolve, or complete, that which was unresolved while he lived. I feel this strongly in my heart.

Einstein once said that either nothing is a miracle, or everything is. To me, everything is. And even now, the little things in life that we usually take for granted still seem miraculous. Each day, when I thank God for being alive, my prayer washes away the problems, the stress, and the trivia all around me, and refocuses me in that moment, in that miracle. I take a deep breath into my new lungs and recall a time when even breathing was difficult.

These days, when I look in the mirror, I don't see old, tired, and blue. I see gray hair, but instead of being distressed by it, I'm elated. For years, I didn't expect to live long enough ever to see signs of normal aging.

The more time goes by, the more integrated my heart and lungs become. I'm now at the point where I sometimes wonder: Did these things really happen to me? I feel so *normal* now.

A couple of years ago I had some surgery that wasn't related to my heart or lungs. Before the operation, a nurse was taking my medical history.

"Any operations?"

"Well, I had my tonsils out as a kid. And a few years ago my spleen was removed."

"Okay, anything else?"

"Not that I can think of," I told her. "Well — I did have a heart-lung transplant in 1988."

"What?!" She tossed her pen in the air and dropped her head on the desk. She must have thought I was crazy, but for a moment I had forgotten all about the transplant.

But I am still aware of how different my life is. These days, when I hear music, I get excited about the next time I'll go dancing, because I know there will *be* a next time. When I was sick, music was a painful reminder of my limitations. Today, it's a cause for hope and gratitude.

I feel privileged to be alive.

Note

Robert Bosnak and I are continuing our research into unusual experiences of organ transplant recipients. We would appreciate hearing from people who are willing to share their stories. Please write us at the Center for Psychology and Social Change, Box 398080, Cambridge MA 02139, or call (617) 354-2499. (The Centcr is an affiliate of the Cambridge Hospital.)